Extended Matching Questions

for MRCOG Part 2

Edited by Maneesh N Singh MRCOG
Clinical Research Fellow
Lancashire Teaching Hospitals Trust
Lancaster

Sarah Vause MD MRCOG
Consultant in Feto-Maternal Medicine
St Mary's Hospital
Manchester

Pierre Martin-Hirsch MD MRCOG
Consultant Gynaecologist
Lancashire Teaching Hospitals Trust
Preston

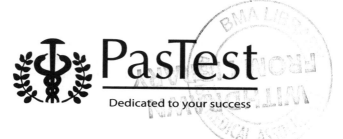

PasTest

Dedicated to your success

© 2007 PASTEST LTD
Egerton Court
Parkgate Estate
Knutsford
Cheshire
WA16 8DX

Telephone: 01565 752000

First published 2007
ISBN: 1 905635 22 2
ISBN: 978 1905635 221

A catalogue record for this book is available from the British Library.

The information contained within this book was obtained by the authors from reliable sources. However, while every effort has been made to ensure its accuracy, no responsibility for loss, damage or injury occasioned to any person acting or refraining from action as a result of information contained herein can be accepted by the publishers or authors.

PasTest Revision Books and Intensive Courses

PasTest has been established in the field of postgraduate medical education since 1972, providing revision books and intensive study courses for doctors preparing for their professional examinations.
Books and courses are available for the following specialties:
MRCGP, MRCP Parts 1 and 2, MRCPCH Parts 1 and 2, MRCPsych, MRCS, MRCOG Parts 1 and 2, DRCOG, DCH, FRCA, PLAB Parts 1 and 2.
For further details contact:
**PasTest, Freepost, Knutsford, Cheshire WA16 7BR
Tel: 01565 752000 Fax: 01565 650264
www.pastest.co.uk   enquiries@pastest.co.uk**

Text prepared by Keytec Typesetting Ltd, Bridport, Dorset
Printed and bound in Athenaeum Press, Gateshead

Exten~ Questions for

~art 2

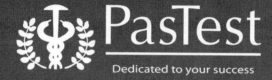

Dedicated to your success

CONTENTS

About the authors   *vii*
Foreword   *ix*
Preface   *xi*
How to Answer EMQs   *xiii*
Abbreviations   *xiv*

QUESTIONS   **1**
Obstetrics   3
Gynaecology   31

ANSWERS   **61**
Obstetrics   63
Gynaecology   83

Index   *101*

ABOUT THE AUTHORS

Maneesh Nandan Singh, MRCOG, is currently working as a clinical research fellow at Lancashire Teaching Hospitals Trust and Lancaster University. His main areas of interest are gynaecological oncology and endometriosis. He is also a member of the MRCOG standard setting committee and is the regional chair of trainees in the North-West Deanery.

Sarah Vause, MD, MRCOG, is currently working as a consultant in feto-maternal medicine at St Mary's Hospital, Manchester. Her interests include cardiac disease in pregnancy.

Pierre Martin-Hirsch, MD, MRCOG, is currently working as a consultant gynaecologist/gynaecological oncologist at Lancashire Teaching Hospitals Trust. His main areas of interest include gynaecological oncology and research methodology. He is also sub-editor for the *British Journal of Obstetrics and Gynaecology* and a contributor to the British Society for Colposcopy and Cervical Pathology (BSCCP) and European guidelines for colposcopy.

FOREWORD

By Professor Anne Garden FRCOG, Director, Centre for Medical Education and Head of Department of Medicine, Lancaster University.

One of the greatest changes that has occurred in the last decade in Medical Education is the emphasis on assessment – designing assessments that are reliable, robust and valid. The increased use of External Matching Questions (EMQs) is part of this welcome change. EMQs allow testing of knowledge in context, applied to clinical scenarios as opposed to mere recall of fact and save us from the temptation of examining minutiae of fact in an attempt to write truly robust questions in the multiple choice format.

To those more accustomed to assessment by essay and multiple choice questions, this can be a major adjustment. I am therefore very pleased to see this book of EMQs published allowing trainees (and maybe a few more mature clinicians who want to test their knowledge is up-to-date!) an opportunity of practising questions in this format. The authors are to be congratulated on writing questions in this format over such a wide range of topics in Obstetrics and Gynaecology. I am sure their readers will have cause to be grateful to them.

PREFACE

Extended matching questions (EMQs) are increasingly being used at both an undergraduate and postgraduate level. The Royal College of Obstetricians and Gynaecologists has recently adopted this method in its Part 2 examination and is about to introduce them into the Part 1 examination.

In the Part 2 examination, EMQs contribute to 15% of the overall mark and may in the future contribute more. At present, MCQs (multiple choice questions) contribute to 25% of the final mark and short answers 60%. At the September 2006 sitting the marks attained by the candidates in the EMQ examination ranged between 50% and 70%.

EMQs have the advantage over MCQs in that they test the applied knowledge of the candidate as well as their factual knowledge. Many of the questions require clinical expertise in order to formulate the correct answer.

This book is intended for candidates preparing for the Part 2 MRCOG examination. The standard of EMQs varies so as to represent the MRCOG examination. All examinations for the MRCOG undergo a formal standard setting procedure and therefore the pass mark will vary according to the difficulty of the exam. This ensures that candidates who pass the exam at one sitting would be expected to pass the exam at any other sitting.

We hope that you find this book helpful in your preparation for the MRCOG and wish you every success.

HOW TO ANSWER EMQs

EMQs consist of four elements: a theme; an option list; a lead in; and a number of stems. The theme is the topic or area being tested, for example 'Emergency gynaecology'. The options consist of the possible answers for the stems. The lead in is the instruction to the candidate, for example 'Choose the most appropriate form of management'. The stems usually consist of the clinical scenario. In the examination be sure to fill in an answer as there is no negative marking for this part. The only negative marking in the whole exam is for persistent factual error in the short question section.

In order to answer the question read the question carefully. Start with the 'lead in' and then move to the stem. The information given in the stems should be sufficient to formulate your own answer. Once you have decided on the answer check the options provided. If your answer is not there, re-read the stem for any information that you have missed and choose the most likely answer from the options. Reading the list of options first is not thought to be helpful as this may distract you and can be time consuming. Clinical obstetrics and gynaecology can be ambiguous, and this ambiguity is reflected in the questions. This can be frustrating for the candidate, but if you follow the principles you will score highly in the examination.

The aim of the questions in this book is to develop the style of answering questions in an efficient manner and also to test your knowledge and clinical expertise.

ABBREVIATIONS

A&E	accident and emergency department
ARM	artificial rupture of membranes
BMI	body mass index
bpm	beats per minute
BRCA	breast cancer gene
CEA	carcinoembryonic antigen
CIN	cervical intraepithelial neoplasia
CT	computed tomography
CTG	cardiotocogram
CVA	cerebrovascular accident
DOA	direct occiput anterior
ECG	electrocardiogram
EMQ	extended matching questions
FSH	follicle-stimulating hormone
hCG	human chorionic gonadotrophin
HPV	human papilloma virus
IUCD	intrauterine contraceptive device
IUGR	intrauterine growth restriction
LBBB	left bundle branch block
LH	luteinising hormone
LOT	left occiput transverse
LSCS	lower segment caesarean section
MRI	magnetic resonance imaging
PCOS	polycystic ovarian syndrome
PCR	polymerase chain reaction
PID	pelvic inflammatory disease
RBBB	right bundle branch block
ROT	right occiput transverse

QUESTIONS

OBSTETRICS

THEME: FETAL WELLBEING

A Deliver immediately
B Do nothing until later in pregnancy
C Ductus venosus Doppler and biophysical profile
D Fetal echo
E Growth scans and liquor volume every 2 weeks
F Kick chart
G Middle cerebral artery peak systolic velocity measurement every week
H Twice weekly cardiotocogram (CTG)
I Uterine artery Doppler

Lead in: For each of the following clinical scenarios please select the most appropriate form of monitoring from the list of options above. Each option may be used once, more than once or not at all.

☐ **1**   A woman has RhD antibody titre of 30 IU/ml. She is currently 24 weeks' gestation. Her last baby required an exchange transfusion in the neonatal period. Her husband is homozygous RhD positive.

☐ **2**   A woman attending a routine antenatal clinic appointment is scanned because the midwife thinks the uterus feels small. She is found to have a fetus with an estimated fetal weight of 590 g at 27 weeks' gestation. There is oligohydramnios and absence of end diastolic flow in the umbilical artery. She has not had steroid injections.

☐ **3**   On an anomaly scan at 20 weeks' gestation a monochorionic diamniotic twin pair appear normal, have normal liquor volumes and are both appropriately grown.

☐ **4**   Gastroschisis is detected on a 20-week anomaly scan. The woman is now 28 weeks pregnant.

THEME: DIABETES IN PREGNANCY

A   Arrange a glucose tolerance test
B   Dietary intervention and blood glucose monitoring
C   Do nothing and review in antenatal clinic
D   Glibenclamide and dietary modification
E   Glucagon
F   Intravenous fluids and sliding scale insulin
G   Metformin and dietary modification
H   Subcutaneous insulin and dietary modification

Lead in: For each of the following clinical situations please select the most appropriate management option from the list above. Each option may be used once, more than once or not at all.

☐   5   A woman with type 2 diabetes is admitted with threatened pre-term labour at 27 weeks' gestation. She is given prophylactic steroids and 18 hours later you are asked to review her because two consecutive blood glucose readings have been 10.3 mmol/l and 12.1 mmol/l.

☐   6   A 37-year-old Asian woman with a body mass index (BMI) of 36 kg/m^2 is referred for a 75 g glucose tolerance test at 28 weeks' gestation. The fasting level is 5.7 mmol/l and the 2-hour level is 7.4 mmol/l.

☐   7   A woman has a glucose tolerance test performed because of a macrosomic baby and polyhydramnios. Her fasting glucose is 8.2 mmol/l and the 2-hour level is 12.4 mmol/l.

☐   8   A professional woman with type 1 diabetes is 12 weeks pregnant. She has extremely tight control. Due to an important business meeting she misses her lunch and collapses at 4 pm.

THEME: HYPERTENSION IN PREGNANCY

A Check platelet count, renal function, clotting and liver function tests
B Enalapril
C Immediate lower segment caesarean section (LSCS)
D Induction of labour
E Labetalol
F Magnesium sulphate, stabilise blood pressure and assess regarding mode of delivery
G Monitor proteinuria and ask the community midwife to check the blood pressure on alternate days
H Sublingual nifedipine

Lead in: For each of the following clinical situations please select the most appropriate management option from the list above. Each option may be used once, more than once or not at all.

☐ **9** You see a primiparous woman in the antenatal clinic who is 38 weeks' gestation. At booking her blood pressure was 110/70 mmHg and last week it was 130/80 mmHg. Today her blood pressure is 145/95 mmHg. She has no proteinuria.

☐ **10** You see a woman at her first hospital antenatal clinic visit. She is 28 weeks' gestation. Her blood pressure is 150/100 mmHg. There is no proteinuria. The woman tells you that she was unable to take the combined oral contraceptive pill because her blood pressure went up when she took it. She is otherwise fit and well. In her hand-held notes her blood pressure was recorded as 150/100 mmHg when she was referred by her general practitioner and 145/95 mmHg when she saw her community midwife 2 weeks ago.

☐ **11** The emergency bell rings. A woman who was being induced for pre-eclampsia at 37 weeks' gestation is fitting. Her blood pressure is 180/100 mmHg. At the last vaginal examination 2 hours ago she was 6 cm dilated.

THEME: ANTI-HYPERTENSIVES IN PREGNANCY

A   α-Blocker
B   β-Blocker
C   Calcium-channel antagonist
D   Centrally acting anti-hypertensive
E   Combined α- and β-blocker
F   Depression
G   Intrauterine growth restriction
H   No proved detrimental effects
I   Palpitations
J   Renal toxicity in the fetus
K   Thiazide diuretic

Lead in: For each of the questions below choose the most appropriate answer from list of options above. Each option may be used once, more than once or not at all.

☐   **12**   A women presents at 12 weeks' gestation with essential hypertension. She is taking a thiazide diuretic. What is the most common risk to the fetus?

☐   **13**   What type of drug is labetalol?

☐   **14**   A 37-year-old woman is started on methyldopa early in pregnancy. She asks you what is its most common side-effect.

☐   **15**   You are called by a general practitioner, who is concerned that a patient of his, who is 7 weeks pregnant, is taking atenolol. He asks you what the risk is to the fetus of prolonged use of atenolol during the pregnancy.

THEME: PRE-ECLAMPSIA

A   Administer furosemide intravenously
B   Administer magnesium sulphate
C   Administer oral labetalol
D   Administer steroids
E   Arrange induction with prostaglandin
F   Calculate mean arterial pressure
G   Commence iv labetalol
H   Continue intravenous Hartmann's solution at the rate of 85 ml/h
I   Immediate iv dose of 10 ml of 10% calcium gluconate
J   Monitor patellar reflexes
K   Obtain iv access
L   Perform caesarean section immediately
M   Provide 500 ml fluid challenge
N   Stop magnesium sulphate
O   Transfer to intensive treatment unit
P   Transfer to postnatal ward

Lead in: For each of the scenarios below choose the most appropriate initial management from the list of options above. Each option may be used once, more than once or not at all.

☐ **16**   A 36-year-old primigravida is admitted from home with severe gestational proteinuric hypertension at 33 weeks' gestation. She has a severe frontal headache and has not felt the fetus move for the past 24 hours. She has 5 beats of clonus.

☐ **17**   A 24-year-old woman delivered 18 hours earlier via a caesarean section because of severe gestational proteinuric hypertension at 36 weeks. A magnesium sulphate infusion had been commenced 24 hours earlier. She has been oliguric for the past 4 hours and her respiratory rate is 5 per minute.

☐ **18**   A 33-year-old primigravida delivered 10 hours earlier and has been oliguric for the past 4 hours. Magnesium sulphate had been commenced 18 hours earlier for severe gestational proteinuric hypertension.

THEME: INFECTIONS IN PREGNANCY

A   Coxsackie virus
B   Cytomegalovirus
C   Hepatitis A
D   Hepatitis B
E   Herpes simplex
F   Human immunodeficiency virus
G   Parvovirus
H   Rubella
I   *Treponema pallidum*
J   Varicella zoster

Lead in: For each of the following scenarios please select the most likely causative infection from the list of options above. Each option may be used once, more than once or not at all.

☐   **19**   A pregnant woman has malaise, myalgia and a high temperature since 2 days. She has also developed a florid vesicular rash. She is admitted to hospital coughing, tachypnoeic and febrile.

☐   **20**   Ventriculomegaly is seen on an ultrasound scan. A positive viral polymerase chain reaction (PCR) is obtained from amniotic fluid. At postmortem intracellular viral inclusions are found in several organs.

☐   **21**   An ultrasound scan reveals a hydropic fetus with a large placenta. Microcephaly is present. During treatment the woman develops a Jarisch–Herxheimer reaction.

☐   **22**   A children's nursery assistant delivers a baby with hepatosplenomegaly and a petechial rash. When the paediatrician measures the baby's head it is below the third centile.

☐   **23**   A woman is admitted to hospital with urinary retention. Vulval ulceration is noted.

☐   **24**   A baby is born with flexion contractures. The paediatrician also notes that the baby has congenital cataracts.

THEME: GENETICS

A 1:1
B 1:2
C 1:4
D 1:20
E 1:40
F 1:80
G Less than 1:100
H 2:3

Lead in: For each of the following scenarios please select the most accurate estimation of risk from the list of options above. Each option may be used once, more than once or not at all.

☐ **25**   Kate's twin brother has cystic fibrosis. Neither Kate nor her parents have cystic fibrosis. What is the chance of her being a carrier?

☐ **26**   Kate is subsequently tested and found to carry the cystic fibrosis gene. She has a 'one night stand' with a Caucasian man and is pregnant. What are the chances of her baby having cystic fibrosis?

☐ **27**   Kelly has homocystinuria. She is not related to the father of her baby. What is the chance of her baby being a carrier of homocystinuria?

☐ **28**   What are the chances of Kelly's baby having homocystinuria?

☐ **29**   Kelly's mother does not have homocystinuria. What is the chance of her being a carrier?

THEME: ANTENATAL SCREENING

A   20-week anomaly scan
B   Amniocentesis
C   Chorion villus biopsy
D   Cordocentesis
E   Doppler of middle cerebral artery
F   No further investigation needed – review in antenatal clinic
G   No further investigation needed – offer termination
H   Nuchal lucency and first trimester biochemistry
I   Second trimester triple test
J   Take maternal blood for PCR amplification of free fetal DNA

Lead in: For each of the following situations please select the most appropriate initial investigation from the list of options above. Each option may be used once, more than once or not at all.

☐ **30** A couple have a 4-year-old child with Down's syndrome. They feel certain that they would not want to have a second child with Down's syndrome. The woman is 23 years old and is 11 weeks' pregnant.

☐ **31** A woman whose previous pregnancies have been affected by RhD haemolytic disease presents at 16 weeks' gestation. She required intrauterine transfusions during her last pregnancy. Her partner is known to be heterozygous for RhD gene.

☐ **32** Anencephaly is diagnosed on a 14-week scan at booking.

☐ **33** A 42-year-old woman presents at 16 weeks' gestation and requests diagnostic testing for Down's syndrome.

☐ **34** On an 18-week scan, choroid plexus cysts, a congenital heart abnormality, exomphalos and bilateral talipes are noted. The woman is adamant that she will not consider terminating the pregnancy.

☐ **35** A man is known to have a 14:21 balanced translocation. His partner attends for her first appointment at 17 weeks' gestation.

☐ **36** A couple are both known to be carriers of the β-thalassaemia gene. They are clear that they would terminate an affected pregnancy. You see them for the first time at 8 weeks' gestation.

☐ **37** A woman has anti-Kell antibodies. Her husband is known to be homozygous Kell positive. She is 28 weeks' gestation.

THEME: RHESUS DISEASE

A Give 250 IU anti-D
B Give 250 IU anti-D and perform Kleihauer's test
C Give 500 IU anti-D
D Give 500 IU anti-D and perform Kleihauer's test
E Give 1500 IU anti-D
F Give 1500 IU anti-D and perform Kleihauer's test
G No need for anti-D prophylaxis

Lead in: For each of the following clinical situations please select the most appropriate treatment option from the list above. Each option may be used once, more than once or not at all.

☐ **38** An RhD-negative woman has an amniocentesis at 16 weeks.

☐ **39** An RhD-negative woman is admitted to hospital with tightenings after her partner has assaulted her. She is 28 weeks' gestation.

☐ **40** An RhD-negative woman has an unsuccessful attempt at external cephalic version at 37 weeks' gestation. She is booked for LSCS at 39 weeks' gestation.

☐ **41** An RhD-negative woman attends hospital with vaginal bleeding at 32 weeks' gestation. She had prophylactic anti-D (1500 IU) 4 weeks previously.

☐ **42** An RhD-negative woman is known to have RhD antibodies. At delivery her antibody titre is 4 IU. She delivers an RhD-positive baby.

☐ **43** An RhD-negative woman attends the gynaecology unit with vaginal bleeding at 11 weeks' gestation. A scan confirms an ongoing intrauterine viable pregnancy.

THEME: TWIN PREGNANCY

A Dichorionic diamniotic
B Monochorionic diamniotic
C Monochorionic monoamniotic

Lead in: For each of the following clinical situations please select the chorionicity of the twins being described from the list of options above. Each option may be used once, more than once or not at all.

☐ **44** The twins are different sexes.

☐ **45** At 20 weeks' gestation twin to twin transfusion syndrome is diagnosed.

☐ **46** On scan at 10 weeks' gestation a lambda sign is seen.

☐ **47** On scan at 10 weeks' gestation one yolk sac and two fetal poles are seen

☐ **48** On scan at 15 weeks' gestation cord entanglement is apparent.

☐ **49** Selective feticide using potassium chloride was performed for a severe neural tube defect in one fetus.

☐ **50** Cleavage of the embryo occurred between day 0 and day 3.

☐ **51** Cleavage of the embryo occurred between day 9 and day 13.

☐ **52** The pregnant woman cried in the antenatal clinic because a well-meaning junior doctor told her that the risk of perinatal mortality associated with her twin pregnancy was approximately 30%.

THEME: FETAL ULTRASOUND ABNORMALITY

A 45,X0
B 47,XX+13
C 47,XX+18
D 47,XX+21
E Beckwith–Wiedemann syndrome
F Meckel–Gruber syndrome
G Myotonic dystrophy
H Pentalogy of Cantrell
I Prader–Willi syndrome
J Triploidy

Lead in: For each of the following ultrasound abnormalities please select the most likely diagnosis from the list of options above. Each option may be used once, more than once or not at all.

☐ **53** On a 20-week scan the fetus is seen to have an atrioventricular septal defect and a large sandal gap.

☐ **54** The fetus is seen to have polyhydramnios and a double bubble at 34 weeks.

☐ **55** Bilateral talipes, rocker bottom feet and a strawberry-shaped head are noted on a 20-week anomaly scan.

☐ **56** A midline facial cleft and holoprosencephaly is noted at 19 weeks.

☐ **57** A symmetrically small fetus and a very large thick placenta are seen on an anomaly scan.

☐ **58** An encephalocele, large multicystic kidneys and oligohydramnios are noted at 17 weeks.

☐ **59** Choroid plexus cysts, overlapping fingers, clenched fists and a congenital heart abnormality are seen on a 20-week scan.

THEME: DRUGS IN PREGNANCY

A   Cleft palate
B   Discoloured deciduous teeth
C   Enlarged right atrium and tricuspid regurgitation
D   Nasal hypoplasia and chondrodysplasia punctata
E   Neonatal irritability or fitting
F   Neonatal respiratory depression
G   Neural tube defect
H   Reduced liquor volume
I   Virilisation of a female fetus

Lead in: For each of the following scenarios please select from the list of options above the complication with which it is most likely to be associated. Each option may be used once, more than once or not at all.

☐ **60**   An epileptic woman conceives while on phenytoin. She is worried about the possibility of fitting and continues to take the phenytoin while waiting for her first hospital appointment at 14 weeks' gestation.

☐ **61**   A woman with severe sciatica during pregnancy takes indometacin regularly for 4 weeks from 28 weeks.

☐ **62**   A woman with a prosthetic heart valve conceives while on warfarin. She has irregular bleeding and does not realise that she is pregnant until she is 14 weeks' gestation.

☐ **63**   A woman with severe congenital heart disease conceives while on captopril. In view of her heart condition a decision is made to continue captopril during pregnancy.

☐ **64**   A woman with a severe bipolar disorder conceives while on lithium.

THEME: LATE TERMINATION OF PREGNANCY

A Cannot offer termination under clause E
B Hysterotomy
C Induction of labour with mifepristone and prostaglandins
D Potassium chloride feticide prior to induction of labour with
     mifepristone and prostaglandins
E Selective feticide using potassium chloride
F Selective feticide using umbilical cord occlusion
G Suction termination of pregnancy

Lead in: For each of the following clinical scenarios please select the most appropriate method of termination of pregnancy from the list of options above. Each option may be used once, more than once or not at all.

☐ **65** Trisomy 18 is diagnosed on amniocentesis. By the time the result is available the woman is 23 weeks' gestation. She requests termination of pregnancy.

☐ **66** A woman presents for the first time to the antenatal clinic at 30 weeks' gestation. Anencephaly is diagnosed on ultrasound scan. She requests termination of pregnancy.

☐ **67** A severe neural tube defect is diagnosed on ultrasound scan at 20 weeks' gestation in one twin of a monochorionic diamniotic twin pair. The other twin appears healthy. The parents want to terminate the twin with the neural tube defect, but do not want to terminate the healthy twin.

☐ **68** On a scan at 28 weeks' gestation, it is noted that the fetus has a missing hand. The parents request termination of pregnancy.

☐ **69** A 15-year-old girl who is pregnant as a result of child abuse presents at 25 weeks' gestation requesting termination of pregnancy. A scan confirms her dates and the fetus appears normal.

THEME: SPINAL ANATOMY

A C5,C6
B C8
C L1,L2
D L3 L4
E L4,L5,S1,S2,S3
F S1
G S2,S3
H S2,S3,S4
I T10
J T2
K T4
L T6
M T8

Lead in: For each of the following situations please select the most appropriate vertebra, nerve root or dermatome from the list of options above. Each option may be used once, more than once or not at all.

☐ **70** In an adult the spinal cord terminates at the level of these vertebrae.

☐ **71** The subarachnoid space terminates at the level of these vertebrae.

☐ **72** Prior to an elective LSCS an anaesthetist gives a spinal anaesthetic. On initial testing the woman is able to sense 'cold' at the level of her umbilicus. Which dermatome is this?

☐ **73** Which dermatome would the anaesthetist like the regional block to reach before the operation is started?

☐ **74** A senior house officer (SHO) checks the biceps tendon reflex in a woman on a magnesium infusion. Which nerve root(s) are being checked?

☐ **75** A pregnant woman with sciatica complains of numbness on the sole of her foot. Which dermatome is this?

☐ **76** An obstetrician gives a pudendal block. What is the nerve root(s) of the pudendal nerve?

THEME: EMERGENCY DRUG TREATMENT

A Adenosine 3 mg
B Adrenaline 0.5 ml of 1:1000
C Adrenaline 1 mg
D Adrenaline 1 ml of 1:10 000
E Aminophylline 300 mg
F Amiodarone 3 mg
G Amiodarone 300 mg
H Atropine 0.3 mg
I Atropine 3 mg
J Ephedrine 3 mg

Lead in: For each of the following emergency situations please select the most appropriate drug from the list of options above. Each option may be used once, more than once or not at all.

☐ **77** Following an epidural top-up a woman becomes hypotensive and the fetus becomes bradycardic. Neither the maternal hypotension nor the fetal bradycardia responds to positioning her in the left lateral position and a bolus of intravenous fluids.

☐ **78** A woman develops facial oedema and an erythematous rash, is wheezy and has difficulty breathing shortly after being given an intravenous dose of antibiotics.

☐ **79** A woman delivered by LSCS 4 days ago collapses on the postnatal ward. The electrocardiogram (ECG) monitor shows sinus rhythm. You are unable to feel a pulse and she is not breathing. No one has given her any drugs as yet.

☐ **80** A visitor has a cardiac arrest in the hospital corridor. Following defibrillation, his pulse returns but he is bradycardic with a pulse rate of 40 bpm.

THEME: ANTENATAL PROBLEMS

A Admit for steroids and arrange induction of labour in 48 hours
B Admit for steroids and delivery within 48 hours by caesarean section
C Artificial rupture of membranes
D Artificial rupture of membranes and commence oxytocin (Syntocinon)
E Daily CTG and repeat Doppler and liquor in 1 week
F Deliver by caesarean section as soon as possible
G Deliver by emergency caesarean section
H Induction of labour with prostaglandin in 1 week
I Induction of labour with Syntocinon
J Induction of labour within 24 hours with prostaglandin
K Perform ultrasound scan on delivery suite
L Repeat Doppler and liquor in 1 week
M Repeat Doppler and liquor in 2 days and administer steroids
N Repeat Doppler and liquor in 24 hours
O Repeat growth scan in 1 week
P Repeat growth scan in 2 weeks

Lead in: For each of the scenarios described below, choose the most appropriate management option from the list above. Each option may be used once, more than once or not at all.

☐ **81** You are asked to see a G1P0 on the antenatal ward at 32 weeks' gestation. She has gestational diabetes and an ultrasound scan has demonstrated growth below the tenth centile and absence of end diastolic flow; the liquor appears normal. The CTG today is normal.

☐ **82** A G2P1 is seen in antenatal clinic at 34 weeks' gestation. She has no other medical problems, and has had a 2.4 kg baby delivered at 38 weeks previously. Ultrasound scan suggests growth is below tenth centile and amniotic fluid index is 5. The Doppler and CTG are both normal.

☐ **83** A 25-year-old G1P0 is seen in antenatal clinic at 37 weeks. She has had an uneventful pregnancy, but has developed some itching of the palms and soles. Bile acids level is 80 µmol/l and alanine aminotransferase (ALT) is 300 iu/l. She has no proteinuria and the presentation is cephalic.

☐ **84** A 36-week G1P0 has prelabour rupture of membranes. She returns from home 12 hours later complaining of a green vaginal discharge. She is afebrile and the CTG is normal. The presentation is cephalic and her Bishop's score is 2.

☐ **85** A 33-week G1P0 has been admitted with a 20 ml vaginal bleed and irregular painful tightenings. She has no antenatal problems. On examination the presentation is cephalic and the fundus measures 30 cm. The CTG demonstrates reduced variability, shallow variable decelerations and a baseline of 160 bpm. The maternal pulse is 80 bpm. The cervix is long and closed.

THEME: MANAGEMENT ON THE DELIVERY SUITE

A Administer dinoprostone gel
B Admit for steroids and arrange caesarean section in 48 hours
C Admit for steroids and delivery within 48 hours by caesarean section
D Admit to antenatal ward and induction of labour with prostaglandin in 1 week
E Admit to antenatal ward and review the next day regarding mode of delivery
F Artificial rupture of membranes
G Artificial rupture of membranes and commence Syntocinon
H Delay induction and review in clinic in 1 week
I Deliver by urgent caesarean section
J Doppler and liquor in 24 hours
K Induction of labour with Syntocinon
L Monitor on delivery suite for fetal or maternal compromise
M Perform elective caesarean section the next day

Lead in: For each of the scenarios described below, choose the most appropriate management option from the list above. Each option may be used once, more than once or not at all.

☐ **86** A 32-year-old woman is brought in by ambulance. She is complaining of a dull right-sided abdominal pain and a moderate loss per vagina (PV) at 32 weeks' gestation. The CTG shows a baseline of 150 bpm and variability of 5 bpm. Maternal pulse is 120 bpm and blood pressure 120/70 mmHg. The cervix is long and closed.

87 A 30-year-old G3P2 attends the delivery suite for induction of labour at 38 weeks' gestation for fetal macrosomia. She has no significant antenatal history and has had some irregular contractions in the past few days. Bishop's score is 2 and there is no presenting part in the pelvis. An ultrasound scan on the delivery suite demonstrates a transverse lie with the fetal back lying cranially.

88 A 40-year-old primigravida attends with a 30 ml PV bleed at 36 weeks' gestation at 6 am. The fetus is in a breech presentation and an ultrasound scan on the delivery suite suggests a placenta praevia. The maternal pulse is 80 bpm and blood pressure 110/75 mmHg. The CTG demonstrates a baseline of 140 bpm with good variability and accelerations.

THEME: BREAST CANCER IN PREGNANCY

A 1 in 3000
B 1 in 5000
C 1 in 10 000
D Advise against future pregnancy as the prognosis is worse
E Advise to wait 2–3 years after treatment of breast cancer
F Advise to wait 5 years after treatment of breast cancer
G If becomes pregnant than termination is warranted

Lead in: For each of the following questions choose the most appropriate answer from the list of options above. Each option may be used once, more than once or not at all.

89 A 34-year-old woman who has had treatment for breast cancer attends a pre-conceptual clinic wanting advice with regard to her prognosis if she has a pregnancy.

90 What is the incidence of breast cancer in pregnancy?

THEME: MALPRESENTATION

A   Do nothing and review in antenatal clinic
B   Elective caesarean section
C   Emergency caesarean section
D   External cephalic version
E   Internal podalic version
F   Vaginal breech delivery

Lead in: For each of the following clinical scenarios please select the most appropriate management option from the list above. Each option may be used once, more than once or not at all.

☐ **91** A multiparous patient is admitted to the delivery suite with irregular tightenings at term. The tightenings have now settled completely but a breech presentation is suspected and confirmed on scan. The cervix is closed and membranes are intact.

☐ **92** You are attending a twin delivery. The first twin delivered normally 10 minutes ago. The second twin is transverse and decelerations are present on the CTG.

☐ **93** In antenatal clinic you diagnose a breech presentation in a woman at 34 weeks' gestation. The woman has had an LSCS previously and is keen to have a normal delivery this time.

☐ **94** You are called by a distressed midwife who has just realised that what she thought was a vertex is actually a breech. The woman is fully dilated and the breech is 2 cm below the ischial spines. She is multiparous, has made good progress in labour, is contracting well and wants to push.

☐ **95** You are asked to review a woman who is 23 weeks' gestation because she is contracting. She ruptured her membranes at 19 weeks' gestation. She has offensive liquor and is pyrexial. Her cervix is 5 cm dilated and the presentation is breech.

THEME: ANTENATAL MANAGEMENT

A   Caesarean section within 24 hours
B   Do nothing and review in antenatal clinic in 1 week
C   Elective caesarean section at term
D   Emergency caesarean section
E   Expectant management and induce only if post-mature
F   Expectant management and perform caesarean section if post-mature
G   Induction of labour as soon as possible
H   Induction of labour at 38 weeks
I   Induction of labour at 40 weeks
J   Induction of labour in 24 hours
K   Repeat growth scan at 38 weeks' gestation
L   Repeat growth scan in 1 week

Lead in: For each of the scenarios described below, choose the most appropriate management option from the list above. Each option may be used once, more than once or not at all.

☐   **96**   In the antenatal clinic you are asked to counsel a 37-week G2P1 who had a fourth degree tear after delivering a 3.8 kg baby previously. The symphysis–fundal height is appropriate and she is otherwise well. She reports normal urinary and faecal functions.

☐   **97**   You are reviewing a primigravida who has had a growth scan with an estimated fetal weight of 4.4 kg at 38 weeks' gestation. The presentation is cephalic and 3/5 of the head is palpable abdominally. Vaginal examination reveals a long and closed cervix.

☐   **98**   You are asked to counsel a G2P1 at 32 weeks' gestation who has had a previous vaginal delivery of a 3.6 kg baby at term complicated by shoulder dystocia. On reviewing the notes you find that she delivered in McRoberts' position with suprapubic pressure.

☐   **99**   You are asked to see a G1P0 with type 1 diabetes who has had an estimated fetal weight at 38 weeks of 4.3 kg. The head is engaged and Bishop's score is 4. Otherwise the pregnancy is uncomplicated and she is keen to have a normal delivery.

☐   **100**   At 28 weeks' gestation a G2P1 is asking about mode of delivery in this pregnancy. The last delivery was complicated by shoulder dystocia involving delivery of the posterior arm.

□ **101** A G2P1 is seen in the antenatal clinic at 41 weeks' gestation. She had a caesarean section at 5 cm dilatation because of failure to progress. She would like to try for a vaginal delivery as she feels she has been robbed of a natural delivery.

THEME: OBSTETRIC COLLAPSE

A Amniotic fluid embolism
B Cardiomyopathy
C Chest infection
D Cerebrovascular accident (CVA)
E Endocarditis
F Myocardial infarction
G Placenta praevia
H Placental abruption
I Pre-eclampsia
J Primary postpartum haemorrhage
K Secondary postpartum haemorrhage
L Sepsis
M Substance misuse
N Thromboembolism
O Urinary tract infection
P Uterine rupture

Lead in: For each of the scenarios described below, choose the most appropriate diagnosis from the list of options above. Each option may be used once, more than once or not at all.

□ **102** A 37-year-old primigravida presents with 50 ml vaginal blood loss and irregular tightenings at 39 weeks' gestation. Antenatally, there have been no complications. On examination, there is mild generalised discomfort and the head is five-fifths palpable.

□ **103** A 30-year-old primigravida collapses 20 minutes after delivery with a blood pressure of 80/40 mmHg. She is afebrile, and oxygen saturation is 80%. There is no abnormal vaginal bleeding.

□ **104** A 38-year-old G5P1 collapses at 32 weeks' gestation. Prior to collapse she complains of left-sided pelvic pain. Despite resuscitation she dies within 15 minutes.

☐ **105** A 35-year-old primigravida presents with 50 ml vaginal blood loss and irregular tightenings at 35 weeks' gestation. Antenatally, there have been no complications. On examination, the symphysis–fundal height is 32 cm. The cervix is closed and the CTG demonstrates a baseline rate of 170 bpm with a beat to beat variability < 5 bpm.

☐ **106** A 30-year-old primigravida presents on the maternity ward with heavy vaginal bleeding 18 hours after a normal delivery. She is cold and clammy and the uterus is palpable 2 cm above the level of the umbilicus.

☐ **107** You are asked to see a 38-year-old G2P1. She is 6 cm dilated, station −2; 15 minutes earlier the CTG showed fetal tachycardia. On repeat vaginal examination there is no presenting part.

THEME: ACUTE PRESENTATION IN OBSTETRICS

A Abruptio placentae
B Appendicitis
C Atonic uterus
D Cervical incompetence
E Fibroid uterus
F Pancreatitis
G Pelvic inflammatory disease
H Placenta praevia
I Premature prelabour rupture of membranes
J Pre-term labour
K Symphysis pubis disorder
L Tissue trauma
M Torsion of an ovarian cyst
N Urinary tract infection
O Uterine inversion
P Vasa praevia

Lead in: For each of the scenarios described below, choose the most appropriate diagnosis from the list of options above. Each option may be used once, more than once or not at all.

☐ **108** A primigravida presents at 24 weeks' gestation complaining of generalised abdominal pain. The uterus feels large for dates. The fetal heart is present and she has no vaginal loss.

☐ **109** You are called to see a collapsed patient on the labour ward who has just delivered her first baby normally. Her blood pressure is 80/40 mmHg and pulse rate is 60 bpm. The estimated blood loss thus far is 150 ml.

☐ **110** You have just delivered the third baby of a woman by vacuum extraction and are writing the delivery in the notes. You are called back urgently as she is bleeding vaginally.

☐ **111** A 22-week primigravida is admitted to the labour ward with left iliac fossa pain. On examination she is febrile and the uterus is soft, however, there is rebound tenderness in the left iliac fossa.

☐ **112** You are asked to see a G1P0 on the labour ward who is being induced for post-maturity. Five minutes earlier, the midwife had carried out artificial rupture of membranes (ARM) at 3 cm, and the liquor was blood-stained. The patient now has profound bradycardia.

THEME: LABOUR WARD MANAGEMENT

A Administer epidural
B Allow 1 hour for head descent
C Apply fetal scalp electrode
D ARM and await events
E ARM and commence Syntocinon
F Call for senior help
G Commence Syntocinon
H Commence Syntocinon and reassess vaginally in 2 hours
I Deliver by caesarean section
J Deliver by Neville–Barnes forceps
K Deliver by vacuum extraction
L Increase rate of Syntocinon and reassess in 4 hours
M Induction of labour with prostaglandin
N Induction of labour with prostaglandin
O Perform fetal blood sample
P Reassess vaginally in 2 hours

Lead in: For each of the scenarios described below, choose the most management option from the list above. Each option may be used once, more than once or not at all.

☐ **113** You are asked to review a G1P0 who has had a long induction with Syntocinon for 14 hours. She has remained at 2 cm dilatation for 10 hours and is using pethidine for pain relief. The CTG is normal. On vaginal examination she is now 6 cm dilated, but she is requesting a caesarean section.

☐ **114** A G3P2 is admitted in spontaneous labour at term. You have been called as she has profound bradycardia and is 6 cm dilated. The decision has been made to perform an emergency caesarean section under general anaesthesia. While administering a catheter under general anaesthesia in theatre the midwife tells you that the fetal head is visible and the patient is fully dilated.

☐ **115** You are asked to review a G1P0 who has been fully dilated for the past 2 hours. The CTG demonstrates prolonged late decelerations, a baseline of 140 bpm and an adequate variability. On vaginal examination the cervix is fully dilated, the head is direct occiput anterior (DOA) and station +2. You explain that you need to perform an instrumental delivery. The patient refuses any form of instrumental delivery.

☐ **116** You are asked to see a G1P0 on the labour ward at 34 weeks' gestation. She has been fully dilated for 90 minutes. The head is DOA and the station +2. She is contracting well and the CTG is non-reassuring.

THEME: MANAGEMENT OF THE SECOND STAGE OF LABOUR

A   Administer epidural
B   Admit to ward
C   Allow 1 hour for head descent
D   Apply fetal scalp electrode
E   Arrange an urgent ultrasound scan
F   Artificial rupture of membranes
G   Call for senior help
H   Deliver by emergency caesarean section
I   Deliver by Neville–Barnes forceps
J   Deliver by vacuum extraction
K   External cephalic version
L   Increase rate of Syntocinon
M   Induction of labour with prostaglandin
N   Internal podalic version
O   Perform fetal blood sample
P   Start Syntocinon

Lead in: For each of the scenarios described below, choose the most appropriate management option from the list above. Each option may be used once, more than once or not at all.

☐ **117** You are called to see a primigravida at term. She has been pushing for 1 hour and has not delivered. Her contractions are 1 in 10 minutes, abdominally 0/5 of the head is palpable. The position of the head is left occiput transverse (LOT) and is at 1+ station and the CTG demonstrates early decelerations with normal variability and no accelerations with a baseline of 150 bpm.

☐ **118** A primigravida has progressed to 6 cm on Syntocinon. She is contracting 1 in 5 minutes and has now not progressed for 4 hours. Syntocinon is running at 24 ml/h. The position of the head is right occiput transverse (ROT) and the station is at the spines.

☐ **119** After delivering the first twin of a dichorionic pregnancy, the second twin is lying in a transverse position. There is no evidence of fetal distress.

THEME: POSTPARTUM HAEMORRHAGE

A Administer carboprost (Hemabate)
B Administer ergometrine with oxytocin (Syntometrine)
C Ask for platelets to be cross-matched
D Atonic uterus
E Call for senior help
F Commence Syntocinon infusion
G Complete hospital incident report
H Convert to general anaesthesia
I Cross-match 4–6 units of blood
J Examine under general anaesthesia
K Insert a B-lynch suture
L Insert intrauterine balloon
M Thrombophilia
N Tissue trauma
O Total abdominal hysterectomy
P Uterine artery embolisation

Lead in: For each of the scenarios described below, choose the most appropriate initial management option from the list above. Each option may be used once, more than once or not at all.

☐ **120** While carrying out a caesarean section under spinal at night in a woman in labour, on opening the peritoneum you notice that the placenta is protruding through the uterine scar.

☐ **121** A woman is bleeding excessively after a normal delivery. Despite an additional dose of Syntometrine and a Syntocinon infusion, the fundus of the uterus is lying above the level of the umbilicus. A unit of blood is currently being infused, and blood loss is continuous.

☐ **122** After delivery of the placenta, a woman is bleeding heavily per vaginam. She has had an active third stage of labour.

THEME: PROBLEMS IN THE PUERPERIUM

A Atonic uterus
B Breast abscess
C Chest infection
D Constipation
E Endometritis
F Exacerbation of asthma
G Intra-abdominal bleed
H Mastitis
I Postnatal depression
J Pre-eclampsia
K Puerperal psychosis
L Retained products of conception
M Return of menses
N Thromboembolism
O Urinary tract infection
P Wound infection

Lead in: For each of the scenarios described below, choose the most appropriate diagnosis from the list of options above. Each option may be used once, more than once or not at all.

☐ **123** A 20-year-old G1P1 is discharged home 5 days after a prolonged labour, failed forceps delivery and caesarean section. She returns complaining of lower abdominal pain. Her temperature is 38.1 °C, and her uterus is tender and palpable at the umbilicus. Lochia appears offensive and heavy. Cervical examination reveals a multiparous os.

☐ **124** You are asked to see a 32-year-old woman who has had an emergency caesarean section 4 days earlier for a prolonged first stage of labour. Her pulse rate is 120 bpm, respiratory rate 20 per minute and temperature 37.5 °C. On auscultation her chest is clear and oxygen saturation is 90% on air.

☐ **125** A 36-year-old woman has returned to the ward after 4 hours in theatre for a caesarean section because of a prolonged first stage of labour. On examination she is pale and clammy. There is a heavy loss vaginally and the uterus is at the level of the umbilicus. She has passed 80 ml of urine in the catheter bag since delivery.

☐ **126** You are asked to see a woman on the postnatal ward. Her temperature is 39 °C. She has had a normal delivery 3 days previously. Her breasts are tender, with the right breast erythematous and markedly tender but not fluctuant. The uterus is just palpable abdominally and the lochia is normal. Urinalysis is negative.

GYNAECOLOGY

THEME: AMBIGUOUS GENITALIA AND PRIMARY AMENORRHOEA

A   Androgen insensitivity
B   Congenital adrenal hyperplasia
C   Constitutional delay
D   Galactosaemia
E   Gonadal dysgenesis
F   Hyperprolactinaemia
G   Hypogonadotrophic hypogonadism
H   Imperforate hymen
I   Kallmann's syndrome
J   Meyer–Rokitansky–Köster–Hauser syndrome
K   Polycystic ovarian disease
L   Premature ovarian failure
M   Transverse vaginal septum
N   True hermaphrodite
O   Turner's syndrome

Lead in: For each of the scenarios described below, choose the most appropriate diagnosis from the list of options above. Each option may be used once, more than once or not at all.

☐ **127** A 16-year-old girl has been referred by the renal physician with an absent kidney. She has normal secondary sexual characteristics, a 46,XX karyotype and normal external genitalia but absent uterus. What is the most likely diagnosis?

☐ **128** A neonate is delivered with ambiguous genitalia. Further evaluation demonstrates the baby to be 46,XY. There is a uterus present on ultrasound examination.

☐ **129** A 15-year-old girl presents with primary amenorrhoea but normal breast development. The uterus is absent, and chromosomal analysis reveals a 46,XY karyotype.

☐ **130** A 15-year-old girl presents with short stature, absence of pubic hair and inadequate breast development. She is also amenorrhoeic.

☐ **131** A 14-year-old girl presents with primary amenorrhoea. She is of normal stature. On close questioning she has anosmia.

THEME: SEXUAL HEALTH

A *Actinomyces israelii*
B *Calymmatobacterium granulomatis*
C *Candida albicans*
D *Chlamydia trachomatis*
E *Gardnerella vaginalis*
F Group B haemolytic streptococcus
G Herpes simplex
H Human papilloma virus
I *Mycobacterium tuberculosis*
J *Neisseria gonorrhoeae*
K *Staphylococcus aureus*
L *Trichomonas vaginalis*

Lead in: For each of the scenarios described below, choose the most likely causative organism from the list of options above. Each option may be used once, more than once or not at all.

☐ **132** A 36-year-old woman, who has recently emigrated from Africa, is complaining of vulval bleeding. On examination extensive 'beefy-red' ulceration is seen. It is not painful.

☐ **133** A 24-year-old woman presents with urinary retention and severe vulval pain. On examination she has numerous small ulcerated lesions.

☐ **134** An 18-year-old is complaining of an irritant vaginal discharge. On examination there is vulval and vaginal erythema and a grey discharge.

☐ **135** At laparoscopy on a 28-year-old woman with pelvic pain, adhesions around the liver are seen.

☐ **136** A 38-year-old who is 14 weeks pregnant is complaining of a non-itchy vaginal discharge. In a previous pregnancy her baby had severe neonatal infection and spent 14 days on the neonatal unit.

☐ **137** A 33-year-old woman undergoes colposcopy and is found to have strawberry spots on the cervix and vagina.

THEME: CONTRACEPTION

A   Combined oral contraceptive pill
B   Copper intrauterine contraception device (IUCD)
C   Depot-Provera
D   GyneFix IUCD
E   Implanon implant
F   Laparoscopic sterilisation
G   Levonelle
H   Levonorgestrel intrauterine system
I   Male contraception
J   Mini-laparotomy and sterilisation
K   Progesterone-only pill
L   Sheath/condom
M   Withdrawal

Lead in: For each of the scenarios described below, choose the most appropriate contraceptive advice from the list of options above. Each option may be used once, more than once or not at all.

☐ **138** A 16-year-old with Eisenmenger's complex consults you for contraceptive advice.

☐ **139** A 42-year-old multiparous single woman with a BMI of 35 consults you for advice regarding contraception. She had a termination 6 months ago while on the combined oral contraceptive pill.

☐ **140** A married 38-year-old P4 requires contraception. She has had all four children by caesarean section. Her BMI is 38 and she has previously had deep vein thrombosis. What form of contraception would you advise?

☐ **141** A 27-year-old nulliparous student is requesting contraception. She refuses any form of hormonal preparation.

THEME: EMERGENCY GYNAECOLOGY (1)

A Appendicitis
B *Candida* infection
C Complete miscarriage
D Constipation
E Ectopic pregnancy
F Endometriosis
G Endometritis
H Gestational trophoblastic disease
I Herpes infection
J Incomplete miscarriage
K Ovarian torsion
L Pelvic inflammatory disease (PID)
M Retained products of conception
N Retroverted uterus
O Threatened miscarriage
P Urinary tract infection

Lead in: For each of the scenarios described below, choose the most appropriate diagnosis from the list of options above. Each option may be used once, more than once or not at all.

☐ **142** A 19-year-old primigravida presents with urinary retention and bilateral loin tenderness at 14 weeks' gestation. On catheterisation she passes 800 ml of urine. Urine dipstick is negative and no abnormalities are detected on examination.

☐ **143** A 24-year-old presents with right-sided abdominal pain. She complains of diarrhoea and a white vaginal discharge. Her temperature is 38.0 °C. On examination she is tender in the right fornix and there are no masses felt. Urine dipstick is negative as is the pregnancy test.

☐ **144** An asymptomatic 30-year-old G2P1 is seen on the early pregnancy unit with a follow-up human chorionic gonadotrophin (hCG) level of 600 IU. Two days previously the hCG level was 450 IU, and 4 days ago the hCG was 500 IU. An ultrasound scan indicated a possible sac in the endometrial cavity.

☐ **145** A 35-year-old woman presents with worsening right iliac fossa pain. She has rebound tenderness in the right iliac fossa, is pyrexial and has a pulse rate of 120 bpm. She has a grid iron scar.

THEME: EMERGENCY GYNAECOLOGY (2)

A   Administer Syntometrine intramuscularly
B   Admit for observation
C   Check β-hCG in 48 hours
D   Diagnostic laparoscopy
E   Give broad-spectrum antibiotics
F   Intramuscular methotrexate
G   Laparoscopic salpingectomy
H   Laparotomy and salpingectomy
I   Medical management of miscarriage
J   Reassure and discharge
K   Refer to regional centre for further treatment
L   Repeat surgical evacuation
M   Repeat ultrasound scan in 7–10 days
N   Surgical evacuation of uterus
O   Ultrasound scan immediately

Lead in: For each of the scenarios described below, choose the most appropriate management option from the list above. Each option may be used once, more than once or not at all.

☐ **146** A 34-year-old P1 had an evacuation of uterus 6 weeks earlier. Histological examination at that time confirmed a molar pregnancy. She now presents with recurrent moderate bleeding per vaginam and an hCG level of 600 IU. An ultrasound scan suggests the possibility of retained products of conception.

☐ **147** A 28-year-old primigravida presents with painless vaginal bleeding. Her hCG level is 900 IU. An ultrasound scan demonstrates an empty uterus, no free fluid and a 4 cm ovarian cyst.

☐ **148** An 18-year-old woman is admitted to A&E with a positive pregnancy test and 4 weeks' amenorrhoea. Her blood pressure is 70/30 mmHg and pulse rate 86 bpm.

☐ **149** A 26-year-old woman is seen in the gynaecology clinic 12 weeks after a laparoscopic salpingectomy for ectopic pregnancy. She remains amenorrhoeic and her pregnancy test is positive. She denies sexual intercourse since her operation. An ultrasound scan shows an empty uterus and her β-hCG is 890 IU.

☐ **150** A 19-year-old is seen on the early pregnancy assessment unit with painless, mild bleeding per vaginam. She has history of 5 weeks' amenorrhoea and a β-hCG level of 638 IU. An ultrasound scan demonstrates a normal pelvis and empty uterus.

☐ **151** A 23-year-old is seen on the early pregnancy assessment unit with heavy bleeding per vaginam. She has history of 12 weeks' amenorrhoea. On examination the cervix is open and products have been removed from the cervical os, but the bleeding continues. Her pulse is 120 bpm and her blood pressure 100/60 mmHg.

THEME: CLINICAL GYNAECOLOGICAL PROBLEMS

A Adenomyosis
B Bacterial vaginosis
C *Candida* infection
D Cervical cancer
E Cervical dysplasia
F Cervical ectopy
G *Chlamydia* infection
H Dysfunctional uterine bleeding
I Endocervical polyp
J Endometrial cancer
K Endometriosis
L Gonococcal infection
M Syphilis
N Urinary tract infection
O Vaginal atrophy
P Vulval cancer

Lead in: For each of the scenarios described below, choose the most appropriate diagnosis from the list of options above. Each option may be used once, more than once or not at all.

☐ **152** A 23-year-old complains of an offensive vaginal discharge when having penetrative sexual intercourse. On examination an offensive discharge is found on bimanual examination.

☐ **153** A 43-year-old woman presents with deep dyspareunia and menorrhagia. The uterus is tender on bimanual examination. At laparoscopy the pelvis is normal.

☐ **154** A 56-year-old woman presents with pruritus vulvae. On examination the vulva is erythematous. Betametasone prescribed by the general practitioner has not proved to be efficacious.

☐ **155** A 36-year-old is complaining of increased malodorous vaginal discharge. Her last smear examination was 6 months ago. No abnormality is found on examination.

THEME: ABNORMAL BLEEDING

A Adenomyosis
B *Candida* infection
C Cervical cancer
D Cervical dysplasia
E Cervical ectopy
F *Chlamydia* infection
G Dysfunctional uterine bleeding
H Endocervical polyp
I Endometrial cancer
J Endometrial hyperplasia
K Endometriosis
L Gonococcal infection
M Lichen sclerosis
N Ovarian cancer
O Vaginal atrophy
P Vulval cancer

Lead in: For each of the scenarios described below, choose the most appropriate diagnosis from the list of options above. Each option may be used once, more than once or not at all.

☐ **156** A 24-year-old presents with irregular bleeding for the past 3 months. Her BMI is 24 and she has been using Depot-Provera for the past 18 months.

☐ **157** A 32-year-old woman is referred with haematuria, menorrhagia and dyschezia.

☐ **158** A 28-year-old presents with ascites, bilateral adnexal masses and pelvic pain. Her Ca-125 is 72 IU. She has no family history of note. Triple swabs have revealed no evidence of infection.

☐ **159** A 43-year-old woman presents with a 6-month history of heavy, more frequent bleeding. On examination there is no abnormality found and hysteroscopy reveals a normal endometrial cavity.

THEME: GYNAECOLOGICAL INVESTIGATION

A Ca-125
B Cervical smear
C Computed tomography (CT) scan
D Diagnostic laparoscopy
E Endometrial Pipelle
F Follicle-stimulating hormone (FSH), luteinising hormone (LH) and oestradiol
G Full blood count
H Inpatient hysteroscopy
I Magnetic resonance imaging (MRI)
J Outpatient hysteroscopy
K Routine ultrasound scan
L Thyroid function tests
M Triple swabs
N Urgent ultrasound
O Urodynamics

Lead in: For each of the scenarios described below, choose the single most useful investigation from the list of options above. Each option may be used once, more than once or not at all.

☐ **160** A 55-year-old woman presents with postmenopausal bleeding. An ultrasound scan shows a normal uterus and ovaries with an endometrial thickness of 5 mm.

☐ **161** A 42-year-old woman presents with an irregular cycle. Her last cervical smear 1 year ago was normal and she has no menorrhagia.

☐ **162** A 43-year-old woman presents to the gynaecology clinic with bilateral complex ovarian cysts, pelvic ascites and a CA125 of 122 i.u.

☐ **163** A 45-year-old woman with human immunodeficiency virus (HIV) infection presents to the gynaecology clinic with inter-menstrual bleeding and occasional post-coital bleeding.

☐ **164** A 27-year-old woman is seen in the gynaecology clinic with a biopsy result of cervical carcinoma. Vaginal examination reveals a barrel-shaped cervix.

THEME: UROGYNAECOLOGY

A Carcinoma of the bladder
B Detrusor overactivity
C Genuine stress incontinence
D Interstitial cystitis
E Mixed stress incontinence and detrusor instability
F Neurogenic bladder
G Overflow incontinence
H Urethral diverticulum
I Urinary tract infection
J Urogenital atrophy
K Vesico-vaginal fistula

Lead in: For each of the scenarios described below, choose the most appropriate diagnosis from the list of options above. Each option may be used once, more than once or not at all.

☐ **165** A 33-year-old woman presents with a 2-year history of recurrent urinary tract infections and post-micturition dribbling. She is now also complaining of pelvic pain and dyspareunia.

☐ **166** A 38-year-old woman presents 3 months after a cone biopsy. She complains of feeling constantly damp vaginally and is having to wear pads continuously.

☐ **167** A 28-year-old woman presents 7 days after a forceps delivery under regional anaesthesia with frequency of urine, voiding small amounts and occasional leakage of urine on coughing. Her labour was prolonged, and it is recorded in the notes that she passed urine prior to discharge.

☐ **168** A 48-year-old woman presents with a 12-month history of nocturia and incontinence. She has to void small quantities of urine regularly.

☐ **169** A 68-year-old woman returns 4 weeks after insertion of a ring pessary for uterovaginal prolapse. She is complaining of suprapubic tenderness, frequency and dysuria.

THEME: ENDOCRINOLOGY

A Androgen insensitivity
B Hyperthyroidism
C Hypogonadotrophic hypogonadism
D Hypothyroidism
E Menopause
F Pituitary adenoma
G Polycystic ovarian disease (PCOS)
H Premature ovarian failure
I Turner's syndrome

Lead in: For each of the follicular phase endocrine profile results given below, choose the most appropriate diagnosis from the list of options above. Each option may be used once, more than once or not at all.

☐ **170** A 33-year-old with FSH 7.0 IU/l (1–20), LH 4 IU/l (1–20), prolactin 1560 mU/l (50–500), oestradiol 140 pmol/l (130–1500), testosterone 2.0 nmol/l (0.2–3.0), sex hormone binding globulin 43 nmol/l (30–75). Pregnancy test negative.

☐ **171** A 42-year-old with FSH 65 IU/l (1–20), LH 55 IU/l (1–20), prolactin 350 mU/l (50–500), oestradiol 80 pmol/l (130–1500), testosterone 0.5 nmol/l (0.2–3.0), sex hormone binding globulin 43 nmol/l (30–75). Pregnancy test negative.

☐ **172** A 27-year-old with FSH < 1 IU/l (1–20), LH < 1 IU/l (1–20), prolactin 35 mU/l (50–500), oestradiol 80 pmol/l (130–1500), testosterone 0.5 nmol/l (0.2–3.0), sex hormone binding globulin 78 nmol/l (30–75). Pregnancy test negative.

☐ **173** A 27-year-old with FSH 4 IU/l (1–20), LH 12 IU/l (1–20), prolactin 135 mu/l (50–500), oestradiol 180 pmol/l (130–1500), testosterone 3.5 nmol/l (0.2–3.0), sex hormone binding globulin 15 nmol/l (30–75). Pregnancy test negative.

THEME: INFERTILITY

A Androgen insensitivity
B Anti-sperm antibodies
C Asherman's syndrome
D Congenital uterine malformation
E Endometriosis
F Hyperprolactinaemia
G Hyperthyroidism
H Hypogonadotrophic hypogonadism
I Hypothyroidism
J Male factor infertility
K PCOS
L Premature ovarian failure
M Tubal disease
N Turner's syndrome
O Uterine fibroids

Lead in: For each of the scenarios described below, choose the most appropriate diagnosis from the list of options above. Each option may be used once, more than once or not at all.

☐ **174** A 37-year-old woman presents with primary infertility. She has a regular cycle, but complains of deep dyspareunia and dyschezia. Her partner has one child from a previous marriage.

☐ **175** A 20-year-old woman presents with primary infertility. She has been amenorrhoeic for the past 6 months. She has a normal stature and secondary sexual characteristics and her BMI is 18. Her partner is 25 years old and has no significant past medical history.

☐ **176** A 32-year-old woman presents with primary infertility for the past 2 years. Her cycle is 7/33–45 and BMI is 35. Her partner, who is 30 years old, is fit and well.

☐ **177** A 35-year-old woman presents with primary infertility. She has been amenorrhoeic for the past 6 months. Her FSH is 65 IU/l, LH 55 IU/l and oestradiol is < 70 pmol/l. Her partner, who is 43 years old, is fit and well.

THEME: INFERTILITY INVESTIGATION

A   CT head
B   Day 2 FSH
C   Day 21 progesterone
D   Free androgen index
E   Hysteroscopy
F   Laparoscopy and dye perturbation
G   Pelvic ultrasound
H   Rubella antibody titre
I   Semen analysis
J   Serum prolactin
K   Thyroid function test
L   Ultrasound scan

Lead in: For each of the scenarios described below, choose the single most useful test from the list of options above. Each option may be used once, more than once or not at all.

☐ **178** A 37-year-old secretary has a 3-year history of primary infertility. She has regular menses, no dysmenorrhoea or dyspareunia. She has no significant past medical history and is a non-smoker. Her partner is a 39-year-old pub landlord.

☐ **179** A 23-year-old woman has been trying to conceive for the last 9 months. She has no significant history and her cycle is 4/28. Her partner has a child from a previous marriage.

☐ **180** A 29-year-old woman presents with secondary infertility. Her last child was delivered normally 4 years ago but delivery was complicated by postpartum haemorrhage requiring suction evacuation for retained products of conception.

☐ **181** A 33-year-old woman presents with infertility. She has previously had an ectopic removed 3 years earlier and is with the same partner. Her periods are regular and she has no other symptoms.

THEME: CONSENT GUIDELINES

A	1 in 5
B	1 in 50
C	1 in 1000
D	1 in 4000
E	1 in 8000
F	1 in 10 000
G	7 in 1000
H	0.04%
I	1.5%
J	0.5%
K	5%
L	8%
M	10%

Lead in: For each of the questions below, choose the most appropriate answer from the list of options above. Each option may be used once, more than once or not at all.

☐ **182** When consenting a patient for total abdominal hysterectomy, what is the quoted death rate?

☐ **183** What is the risk of ureteric injury when performing total abdominal hysterectomy?

☐ **184** What is the risk of needing a blood transfusion for haemorrhage?

THEME: CONSENT GUIDELINES FOR DIAGNOSTIC LAPAROSCOPY AND VAGINAL HYSTERECTOMY

A	1 in 10
B	1 in 200
C	1 in 50 000
D	1 in 10 000
E	2 in 100
F	2 in 1000
G	5 in 1000
H	5 in 100 000
I	7 in 1000
J	1%
K	4%

Lead in: For each of the questions below, choose the most appropriate answer from the list of options above. Each option may be used once, more than once or not at all.

☐ **185** What is the risk of death from diagnostic laparoscopy?

☐ **186** When consenting a woman for diagnostic laparoscopy, what is the overall risk of serious complications?

☐ **187** When consenting a woman for vaginal hysterectomy, what is the risk of requiring a blood transfusion?

THEME: SURGICAL COMPLICATIONS

A Bleeding requiring resuturing
B Bowel perforation
C Chest infection
D Constipation
E CVA
F Myocardial infarction
G Paralytic ileus
H Pulmonary embolism
I Pulmonary oedema
J Retained swab
K Small-bowel obstruction
L Ureteric injury
M Urinary retention
N Urinary tract infection
O Vault haematoma
P Wound infection

Lead in: For each of the scenarios described below, choose the most appropriate diagnosis from the list of options above. Each option may be used once, more than once or not at all.

☐ **188** A 43-year-old woman presents with generalised abdominal pain and vomiting 11 days after a total abdominal hysterectomy. On examination the abdomen appears distended.

☐ **189** A 66-year-old woman complains of sudden-onset chest pain and shortness of breath 12 hours after pelvic clearance and omentectomy for an ovarian mass. ECG findings reveal acute left bundle branch block (LBBB).

☐ **190** A 41-year-old woman is seen with tachycardia of 140 bpm and some increasing abdominal discomfort following an oophorectomy 4 hours earlier. She appears pale and clammy, but is normotensive.

☐ **191** A 37-year-old woman returns to the gynaecology ward 48 hours after a laparoscopy for pelvic pain. The pain had settled before discharge, but she has been experiencing increasing abdominal pain for the past few hours. Her temperature is 37.9 °C and pulse 100 bpm.

THEME: LAPAROSCOPIC ENTRY TECHNIQUES

A	0.05%
B	0.5%
C	5%
D	10%
E	20%
F	35%
G	50%
H	80%
I	Reduces incidence of bowel and vascular trauma only
J	Reduces incidence of vascular trauma only
K	Reduces incidence of bowel trauma only

Lead in: For each of the questions below, choose the most appropriate answer from the list of options above. Each option may be used once, more than once or not at all.

☐ **192** Bowel adhesions to the anterior abdominal wall are found in what percentage of patients without prior surgery?

☐ **193** What is the advantage of open laparoscopy?

THEME: DRUG THERAPY IN GYNAECOLOGY

A Ampicillin
B Azithromycin
C Cephalexin
D Cephalexin and metronidazole
E Cephalexin, metronidazole and doxycycline
F Clindamycin
G Co-amoxiclav
H Danazol
I Doxycycline
J Duloxetine
K Erythromycin
L Gonadotrophin-releasing hormone analogue
M Mefenamic acid
N Metronidazole
O Tolterodine
P Tranexamic acid

Lead in: For each of the scenarios described below, choose the most likely therapeutic agent responsible for or used in the scenarios above. Each option may be used once, more than once or not at all.

☐ **194** A 38-year-old woman has presented in A&E with shortness of breath, tachycardia and oxygen saturation of 88%. She has recently started taking tablets for menorrhagia.

☐ **195** A swab result from a patient in your gynaecology clinic has demonstrated the presence of *Trichomonas vaginalis*.

☐ **196** A 53-year-old woman has genuine stress incontinence on a recent urodynamics assessment. She does not want surgery.

☐ **197** A 19-year-old girl has had a pregnancy terminated. This is her second termination in 6 months. She was previously treated for a *Chlamydia* infection at her last visit and a recent swab has shown she still has *Chlamydia*.

☐ **198** A pregnant woman is group B haemolytic streptococcus positive. She is allergic to penicillin.

THEME: GYNAECOLOGICAL ONCOLOGY – CERVIX

A   Bilateral salpingo-oophorectomy
B   Chemo-radiation
C   Chemotherapy
D   Colposcopy
E   Cryotherapy
F   CT scan
G   Cytology
H   Laser ablation
I   Loop excision of the transformation zone
J   MRI
K   Pelvic lymph node dissection
L   Punch biopsy
M   Radical hysterectomy
N   Total hysterectomy
O   Trachelectomy
P   Ultrasound scan

Lead in: For each of the scenarios described below, choose the most appropriate management option from the list above. Each option may be used once, more than once or not at all.

☐ **199** A 25-year-old nulliparous woman sees her general practitioner, having had one borderline cervical smear. What is the recommended management?

☐ **200** A 49-year-old multiparous woman sees her colposcopist having had one loop excision which demonstrates CIN3 with incomplete excision margins at the endocervical margin. What is the recommended management?

☐ **201** A 25-year-old nulliparous woman is referred to a gynaecological oncologist with a 1 cm squamous carcinoma of the cervix. What is the optimal imaging technique?

☐ **202** A 30-year-old nulliparous woman is referred to a gynaecological oncologist with a 5 cm squamous carcinoma of the cervix. What further treatment is required?

☐ **203** A 25-year-old nulliparous woman is referred to a gynaecological oncologist with a 1 cm squamous carcinoma of the cervix. She wants to conserve fertility.

THEME: ENDOMETRIAL CANCER

A Aromatase inhibitor
B Chemo-radiation
C Chemotherapy
D Combined contraceptive pill
E CT scan
F Endometrial biopsy
G Herceptin
H Hysteroscopy
I MRI
J Para-aortic node dissection
K Radical hysterectomy
L Smoking
M Tamoxifen
N Total hysterectomy+ bilateral salpingo-oophorectomy
O Trachelectomy
P Ultrasound scan

Lead in: For each of the questions below, choose the most appropriate answer from the list of options above. Each option may be used once, more than once or not at all.

☐ **204** A 45-year-old woman with a recent history of breast cancer is currently taking treatment which puts her at risk of uterine cancer. What is the treatment most likely increasing her risk?

☐ **205** A 57-year-old woman is diagnosed with endometrial cancer. How would you stage her disease?

☐ **206** A 31-year-old woman with a long history of oligomenorrhoea secondary to polycystic ovaries should be advised to take which drug?

THEME: VULVAL NEOPLASIA

A Chemo-radiation
B Combined contraceptive pill
C CT scan
D External beam radiotherapy
E Hysteroscopy
F MRI
G Para-aortic node dissection
H Pelvic lymph node dissection
I Radical vulvectomy
J Sentinel lymph node biopsy
K Smoking
L Superficial and deep ilio-femoral node dissection
M Superficial ilio-femoral node dissection
N Ultrasound scan
O Vulval biopsy
P Wide local excision

Lead in: For each of the questions below, choose the most appropriate answer from the list of options above. Each option may be used once, more than once or not at all.

☐ **207** What is the investigation of choice in a 75-year-old woman with persistent vulval irritation and ulcerated vulval skin?

☐ **208** Which type of lymph node dissection should be undertaken for 3 cm wide squamous vulval carcinoma with a depth of 4 mm?

☐ **209** Which diagnostic procedure might reduce the morbidity associated with groin node dissection?

THEME: VULVAL DISEASE

A Candidal vulvovaginosis
B Condyloma
C Fibroma
D Herniae
E Hidradenitis suppurativa
F Lichen planus
G Lichen sclerosus
H Psoriasis
I Sebaceous cyst

Lead in: For each of the scenarios described below, choose the most appropriate diagnosis from the list of options above. Each option may be used once, more than once or not at all.

☐ **210** A 58-year-old woman presents with a generalised smooth erythematous rash and a history of pruritus vulvae.

☐ **211** An Afro-Caribbean woman presents with chronic painful nodules in the labia majora.

☐ **212** A woman with chronic vulval irritation and a history of diabetes presents to the gynaecology clinic.

THEME: OVARIAN NEOPLASIA

A   Ca-125
B   Carcinoembryonic antigen (CEA)
C   CT scan
D   Endometrioid
E   Interval debulking surgery
F   Mucinous
G   Multiparity
H   Omentectomy
I   Ovulation induction
J   PID
K   Platinum-based chemotherapy
L   Radiotherapy
M   Sensitivity
N   Serous papillary
O   Specificity
P   Ultrasound

Lead in: For each of the questions below, choose the most appropriate answer from the list of options above. Each option may be used once, more than once or not at all.

☐   **213** Which predisposing factor is associated with an increased risk of ovarian cancer?

☐   **214** Which tumour marker might be useful in a 70-year-old woman with suspected Krukenberg's tumour?

☐   **215** Ovarian cancer screening is associated with a high false-positive rate; this is commonly known as low . . . . ?

THEME: CERVICAL CANCER AND DYSKARYOSIS

A	16%
B	30%
C	70%
D	95%
E	Adenocarcinoma
F	Chemoradiation
G	Human papilloma virus (HPV) types 16 and 18
H	HPV types 31 and 33
I	HPV types 6 and 11
J	Interval debulking surgery
K	Menorrhagia
L	Platinum-based chemotherapy
M	Pre-term labour
N	Sensitivity
O	Specificity
P	Squamous carcinoma

Lead in: For each of the questions below, choose the most appropriate answer from the list of options above. Each option may be used once, more than once or not at all.

☐ **216** A 42-year-old woman is treated for stage 1a cervical cancer. She asks what the 5-year survival rate is.

☐ **217** A prophylactic vaccine that protects against genital warts needs to protect against which HPV subtypes?

☐ **218** What is the sensitivity of cervical cytology for mass screening in the UK?

☐ **219** Traditional treatment of cervical intraepithelial neoplasia (CIN) by knife conisation is associated with which complication?

THEME: GESTATIONAL TROPHOBLASTIC DISEASE

A α-fetoprotein
B Ca-125
C Denmark
D CEA
E India
F Copper IUCD
G Chest X-ray
H Chile
I hCG
J Hong Kong
K Mexico
L MRI
M Platinum-based chemotherapy
N UK
O Ultrasound

Lead in: For each of the questions below, choose the most appropriate answer from the list of options above. Each option may be used once, more than once or not at all.

☐ **220** Choriocarcinoma is most common in which country?

☐ **221** A woman presents with persistent vaginal bleeding 8 weeks after a full term delivery and a pelvic mass. Which tumour marker would be most appropriate?

THEME: FAMILIAL AND DRUG-RELATED RISK OF CANCER

A Breast cancer
B Cervical cancer
C Choriocarcinoma
D Endometrial cancer
E Krukenberg's tumour
F Ovarian cancer
G Teratoma
H Vulval cancer

Lead in: For each of the questions below, choose the most appropriate answer from the list of options above. Each option may be used once, more than once or not at all.

☐ **222** A woman presents with a history of risk of hereditary non-polyposis colon cancer. Which gynaecological cancer is she at risk of?

☐ **223** A 30-year-old woman with mutations in the *BRCA1* gene is at risk of which gynaecological cancer?

☐ **224** Women with vulval dystrophy are at risk of which gynaecological cancer?

THEME: GYNAECOLOGICAL ONCOLOGY SURGERY

A Apronectomy
B Cone biopsy
C Ilio-femoral nodes
D Infra-colic omentectomy
E Interval debulking surgery
F Loop excision
G Obturator nodes
H Saphenous vein
I Trachelectomy
J Utero-sacral ligaments
K Vaginal hysterectomy

Lead in: For each of the questions below, choose the most appropriate answer from the list of options above. Each option may be used once, more than once or not at all.

☐ **225** A woman who has completed her family and has incompletely excised cervical glandular intraepithelial neoplasia could undergo which procedure?

☐ **226** Pelvic lymphadenectomy should include which chain of nodes?

☐ **227** A full staging laparotomy for metastatic ovarian cancer should include which procedure?

THEME: CERVICAL SCREENING AND HPV

A   Acetic acid
B   Aciclovir cream
C   Colposcopy
D   HPV testing
E   Imiquimod
F   Laser ablation
G   Liquid-based cytology
H   Loop excision
I   Monsel's solution
J   Pap smear

Lead in: For each of the scenarios described below, choose the most appropriate diagnosis from the list of options above. Each option may be used once, more than once or not at all.

☐   **228**   A postmenopausal woman presents with a type 3 transformation zone on colposcopy with a high grade smear. What treatment should she have?

☐   **229**   Reduction in the number of inadequate cervical smear referrals can be achieved with which test?

☐   **230**   A 25-year-old woman presents to the genitourinary medicine clinic with vulval warts. How is this best managed?

THEME: STATISTICS (1)

A   High sensitivity
B   High specificity
C   High threshold
D   Linear regression
E   Low threshold
F   Negatives verified
G   Pie chart
H   Receiver operator characteristic curve

Lead in: For each of the questions below, choose the most appropriate answer from the list of options above. Each option may be used once, more than once or not at all.

☐ **231** How can you describe a screening test that is very good at detecting disease?

☐ **232** To increase the sensitivity of endometrial thickness measurement in the triage of postmenopausal bleeding do you set a low or high threshold?

☐ **233** A screening test performance across different thresholds is measured by which plot?

THEME: STATISTICS (2)

A Average
B Historical controlled observational study
C Intention to treat analysis
D Meta-analysis
E Narrative review
F Power calculation
G Randomised controlled trial
H Relative risk
I Secondary analysis
J Systematic review

Lead in: For each of the questions below, choose the most appropriate answer from the list of options above. Each option may be used once, more than once or not at all.

☐ **234** You have designed a chemotherapy trial that excludes all the patients who developed side effects and therefore did not complete therapy. What is this described as?

☐ **235** The sample size of a study is assessed by which calculation?

☐ **236** Reliable evidence of clinical practice should be derived from which type of evidence?

☐ **237** A chemotherapy trial that includes all the patients who started the trial is described as what type of analysis?

THEME: STATISTICS (3)

A 6%
B 8%
C 18%
D 33%
E 50%
F 75%
G 87%
H 92%

Lead in: Some bored post-Membership registrars recently conducted a study to determine how well abdominal palpation performed as a screening test for breech presentation. After palpating a woman's abdomen she was then scanned to determine the presentation.

Table 1

	Palpates breech	Palpates cephalic	Total
Scan shows breech	24	8	32
Scan shows cephalic	48	320	368
Total	72	328	400

Lead in: For each of the following questions, select the best estimate from the list of options above. Each option may be used once, more than once or not at all.

☐ **238** What is the prevalence of breech presentation in this population?

☐ **239** What is the sensitivity of abdominal palpation for detecting breech presentation?

☐ **240** What is the specificity of abdominal palpation?

☐ **241** What is the positive predictive value of abdominal palpation for breech presentation?

THEME: ETHICAL AND MEDICO-LEGAL PRINCIPLES

A   Autonomy
B   Battery
C   Beneficence
D   Bolam test
E   Confidentiality
F   Fidelity
G   Fraser (Gillick) competence
H   Negligence
I   Non-maleficence
J   Paternalism
K   Veracity

Lead in: For each of the scenarios described below, choose the most applicable principle from the list of options above. Each option may be used once, more than once or not at all.

☐   **242** A 35-year-old woman is attended by a doctor in labour ward. There is fetal distress, and the doctor performs a forceps delivery. The woman is stressed and communication is difficult, but the doctor proceeds with the forceps delivery.

☐   **243** A midwife repeatedly calls a registrar to attend a G2P1 in prolonged labour. There is a fetal tachycardia and with late decelerations. The doctor eventually arrives, 1 hour after initially being paged. Unfortunately, the baby has cerebral palsy.

☐   **244** A 14-year-old girl presents to clinic requesting termination of pregnancy. She does not want her parents to know that she is having a termination.

☐   **245** A 21-year-old woman undergoes a laparotomy for an ectopic pregnancy. She cancels a holiday due to illness. Six weeks later you receive a letter from an insurance company asking you to write a detailed report that led to the cancellation.

☐   **246** A 68-year-old woman attends for a laparotomy for a suspected endometrial tumour. Her family asks that you do not disclose the diagnosis to the patient as this may affect her psychological wellbeing.

☐ **247** A 45-year-old lady has been diagnosed with fibroids and you decide the best option for her is a hysterectomy.

☐ **248** A Jehovah's witness has an elective caesarean section for a placenta praevia. Despite being counselled about the risks, she wishes not to have a blood transfusion under any circumstance. Despite timely management, the patient dies on the table during a caesarean hysterectomy.

☐ **249** An 18-year-old woman is seen on the antenatal ward collapsed and unconscious with a suspected pulmonary oedema. A caesarean section is performed and the patient survives.

☐ **250** An 83-year-old lady undergoes a laparotomy for suspected ovarian cancer. The family asks to speak to you and asks if you would disclose the results to them first.

ANSWERS

OBSTETRICS

FETAL WELLBEING

1 G – MIDDLE CEREBRAL ARTERY PEAK SYSTOLIC VELOCITY MEASUREMENT EVERY WEEK

Assuming that her husband is the father of the fetus, it is extremely likely that this fetus will become anaemic during this pregnancy. Peak systolic velocity in the middle cerebral artery correlates with the severity of fetal anaemia.

2 C – DUCTUS VENOSUS DOPPLER AND BIOPHYSICAL PROFILE

At 590 g the fetus is small but potentially viable. It is likely that this fetus will require delivery within the next few days. However, there is benefit in attempting to delay delivery until steroids have been administered. Ductus venosus Doppler and biophysical profile would be the best way of assessing fetal reserve and detecting any impending deterioration in fetal condition.

3 E – GROWTH SCANS AND LIQUOR VOLUME EVERY 2 WEEKS

In monochorionic diamniotic twins there is a risk of twin to twin transfusion syndrome. This is diagnosed by discrepancy in liquor volumes in the twins. There is often an associated discrepancy in size.

4 E – GROWTH SCANS AND LIQUOR VOLUME EVERY 2 WEEKS

Fetuses with gastroschisis are at risk of intrauterine growth retardation. Answer E is the most appropriate option from the list (although some may argue that scans could be performed less frequently, every 3 or 4 weeks)

DIABETES IN PREGNANCY

5 F – INTRAVENOUS FLUIDS AND SLIDING SCALE INSULIN

Administration of steroids causes temporary hyperglycaemia. Glycaemic control is best achieved using a sliding scale insulin infusion for 24–48 hours.

6 C – DO NOTHING AND REVIEW IN ANTENATAL CLINIC

These are normal results for a 75 g glucose tolerance test (World Health Organization (WHO) criteria).

7 H – SUBCUTANEOUS INSULIN AND DIETARY MODIFICATION

These results are abnormally high. It is likely that dietary modification alone would be insufficient and that subcutaneous insulin will be needed.

8 E – GLUCAGON

The collapse is likely to be due to hypoglycaemia. Although hypoglycaemia can be averted by glucose drinks or glucose tablets, glucagon injections may be needed in a collapsed patient.

HYPERTENSION IN PREGNANCY

9 G – MONITOR PROTEINURIA AND ASK THE COMMUNITY MIDWIFE TO CHECK THE BLOOD PRESSURE ON ALTERNATE DAYS

At present this patient has non-proteinuric pregnancy-induced hypertension. Therefore she does not have pre-eclampsia and no intervention is required. However, pre-eclampsia could develop. Therefore monitoring for proteinuria is appropriate.

10 E – LABETALOL

This woman appears to have chronic hypertension, not pre-eclampsia. From the available options, treatment with labetalol is the most appropriate. Enalapril, an angiotensin-converting enzyme (ACE) inhibitor, is contra-indicated in pregnancy. Although long-acting nifedipine may be appropriate, sublingual nifedipine could cause a precipitous fall in blood pressure.

11 F – MAGNESIUM SULPHATE, STABILISE BLOOD PRESSURE AND ASSESS REGARDING MODE OF DELIVERY

Prior to delivery this woman requires magnesium sulphate to reduce the risk of further convulsions and stabilisation of her blood pressure. To reduce maternal risks, she should be stabilised prior to anaesthesia. Once she is sufficiently stable the most appropriate route of delivery can be decided. As she is already 6 cm dilated there is a chance that she could be fully dilated and instrumental vaginal delivery performed. If she is not fully dilated delivery should be expedited by LSCS.

ANTI-HYPERTENSIVES IN PREGNANCY

12 H – NO PROVED DETRIMENTAL EFFECTS

There are no proved risks to the fetus with thiazide diuretics. However, it has been postulated that use of diuretics leads to loss of sodium and water and this in turn results in a reduction in blood volume. This directly antagonises a normal physiological process and thus is detrimental to the pregnancy.

13 E – COMBINED α- AND β-BLOCKER

Labetalol is a α- and β-blocker with a low side-effect profile.

14 F – DEPRESSION

Methyldopa is a centrally acting anti-hypertensive, and it can take a few days to achieve hypertensive control. The most common side-effects of methyldopa are depression and tiredness, and occasionally liver dysfunction. Because of the low side-effect profile of labetalol and its speed of action its use is becoming more common.

15 G – INTRAUTERINE GROWTH RESTRICTION

The risks of β-blockers include intrauterine growth restriction. Patients with no other option than to take β-blockers should be scanned serially for growth restriction.

PRE-ECLAMPSIA

16 K – OBTAIN IV ACCESS

The patient has arrived from home. The first concern is always ABC resuscitation and therefore intravenous access is the priority. Stabilisation with magnesium sulphate and anti-hypertensives (if required) followed by delivery is paramount.

17 N – STOP MAGNESIUM SULPHATE

This history is suggestive of magnesium overdose and therefore the first step would be to stop the magnesium sulphate infusion followed by calcium gluconate. Loss of reflexes is a sign that there may be magnesium overdose and this occurs prior to respiratory depression. Magnesium sulphate is preferable to diazepam and phenytoin in reducing the incidence of further fits as it is associated with significant reduction in the need for maternal ventilation, less pneumonia and fewer intensive care admissions. It acts as a membrane stabiliser and reduces intracerebral ischaemia.

18   H – CONTINUE INTRAVENOUS HARTMANN'S SOLUTION AT THE RATE OF 85 ML/H

Oliguria following delivery in severe pre-eclampsia is fairly common. Most units advocate continuing with the fluid regimen for up to 8 hours as there is a risk of pulmonary oedema. Furosemide should not be used until a confirmed diagnosis of pulmonary oedema. Magnesium sulphate is renally excreted. Toxicity is detected by the absence of patellar reflexes, but ultimately respiratory arrest and muscle paralysis or cardiac arrest occur. The antidote is 10 ml of 10% calcium gluconate.

INFECTIONS IN PREGNANCY

19   J – VARICELLA ZOSTER

Varicella zoster (chickenpox) manifests as a vesicular rash. In pregnancy a viral pneumonia can be a serious maternal complication. The incubation period is 14–21 days. The rash is commonly on the face and trunk and minimal on the extremities. Patients are contagious 2 days before the rash until the vesicles have crusted over. Complications in adults include pneumonia, encephalitis and hepatitis. Oral aciclovir can be used in women over 20 weeks' gestation who present within 24 hours of the onset of a rash.

20   B – CYTOMEGALOVIRUS

Viral inclusions can be seen in both parvovirus and cytomegalovirus infections. Congenital cytomegalovirus infection affects the central nervous system and causes ventriculomegaly, whereas parvovirus does not. The rate of primary cytomegalovirus infection is 1–4% and it carries a 40% risk of fetal transmission. The incidence of congenital infection varies between 0.3% and 3%; of these 5% will be symptomatic at birth, with 30% neonatal mortality and long-term morbidity in the majority of survivors. This includes neurodevelopmental delay in up to 90% and hearing loss in 60%.

21   I – *TREPONEMA PALLIDUM*

The ultrasound features are suggestive but not diagnostic of congenital syphilis. A Jarisch–Herxheimer reaction specifically occurs when syphilis is treated with penicillin.

22 B – CYTOMEGALOVIRUS

Congenital cytomegalovirus causes low platelet count and a petechial rash may be seen. Microcephaly may also be a feature.

23 E – HERPES SIMPLEX

Herpes simplex can cause urinary retention. Primary herpes simplex infection has been associated with spontaneous abortion, stillbirth, intrauterine growth restriction and pre-term labour. Management should involve the genitourinary physician, and aciclovir may be used. There is no laboratory or clinical evidence of maternal or fetal toxicity. Use in the last 4 weeks of pregnancy may prevent recurrence of primary herpes in pregnancy.

24 J – VARICELLA ZOSTER

These are feature of congenital varicella syndrome which affects 1–3% of babies of women who develop varicella in pregnancy.

GENETICS

25 H – 2:3

As Kate and her brother are twins there is no doubt about paternity. Cystic fibrosis is an autosomal recessive condition therefore both her mother and father must be carriers. There was a 1:4 chance of her being affected, 1:4 of her not being a carrier and 2:4 of her being a carrier. However we know that she is not affected, which means there is a 2:3 chance of her being a carrier.

26 F – 1:80

The carrier frequency in Caucasians is 1:20. We now know that Kate is a carrier and that if she met another carrier there would be a 1:4 chance of their baby being affected. This gives an overall risk of 1:80 for Kate and her 'one night stand'.

27 A – 1:1

Kelly has two recessive homocystinuria genes. She will definitely pass one of them on to her baby, although it is likely that it will inherit a normal gene from its father. Her baby will certainly be a carrier.

28   G – LESS THAN 1:100

It is unlikely that Kelly's partner will carry the homocystinuria gene. Although the baby will certainly have one recessive gene it is unlikely that it would have two recessive genes, i.e. very unlikely that it is affected.

29   A – 1:1

Both of Kelly's parents must be a carrier of homocystinuria.

ANTENATAL SCREENING

30   C – CHORION VILLUS BIOPSY

The couple have a 1:100 chance of having another baby with Down's syndrome. Screening tests would be inappropriate. Chorion villus biopsy can be offered from 10+ weeks' gestation.

31   J – TAKE MATERNAL BLOOD FOR PCR AMPLIFICATION OF FREE FETAL DNA

There is a 50:50 chance that this fetus is RhD positive, and at risk of being affected. The blood group of the fetus can be ascertained by amplifying free fetal DNA from the maternal circulation. If RhD positive DNA is amplified, this must have come from the fetus as the mother is RhD negative. This test can be done from 16 weeks' gestation.

32   G – NO FURTHER INVESTIGATION NEEDED – OFFER TERMINATION

A conclusive diagnosis of anencephaly can be made at 14 weeks' gestation. The prognosis is lethal. No further investigations are indicated and termination should be offered.

33   B – AMNIOCENTESIS

As the patient has requested diagnostic testing, screening tests are not appropriate. Amniocentesis can be performed from 15 weeks' gestation.

34   F – NO FURTHER INVESTIGATION NEEDED – REVIEW IN ANTENATAL CLINIC

Further investigation will not affect the woman's decision at this stage. It is likely that the fetus has trisomy 18. If the fetus survives until term, the issues may need to be revisited later in pregnancy to plan care around the time of delivery.

35   B – AMNIOCENTESIS

There is a chance that this fetus may have an unbalanced translocation. This can be detected by amniocentesis.

36   C – CHORION VILLUS BIOPSY

There is a 1:4 chance of an affected fetus. Chorion villus biopsy would be the most appropriate initial investigation but could not be performed until 10+ weeks' gestation.

37   E – DOPPLER OF MIDDLE CEREBRAL ARTERY

As the husband is homozygous the fetus will be Kell positive and therefore potentially affected (assuming paternity). Peak systolic velocity in the middle cerebral artery correlates with the degree of anaemia in the fetus.

RHESUS DISEASE

38   A – GIVE 250 IU ANTI-D

Prior to 20 weeks 250 IU anti-D should be given. Kleihauer's test is not necessary.

39   D – GIVE 500 IU ANTI-D AND PERFORM KLEIHAUER'S TEST

After 20 weeks 500 IU anti-D should be given and Kleihauer's test done to see whether this is sufficient. Further doses may be needed if the test indicates a large feto-maternal bleed.

40   D – GIVE 500 IU ANTI-D AND PERFORM KLEIHAUER'S TEST

After 20 weeks 500 IU anti-D should be given and Kleihauer's test done to see whether this is sufficient.

41   B – GIVE 500 IU ANTI-D AND PERFORM KLEIHAUER'S TEST

After 20 weeks 500 IU anti-D should be given and Kleihauer's test done to see whether this is sufficient. This should be done irrespective of whether a routine prophylactic dose has been given recently.

42 G – NO NEED FOR ANTI-D PROPHYLAXIS

This woman is already sensitised. It is too late to give prophylaxis.

43 G – NO NEED FOR ANTI-D PROPHYLAXIS

The Royal College of Gynaecologists (RCOG) green top guidelines suggest that for threatened miscarriage at less than 12 weeks' gestation anti-D is not needed.

TWIN PREGNANCY

44 A – DICHORIONIC DIAMNIOTIC

The twins must be dizygotic and therefore will be dichorionic diamniotic.

45 B – MONOCHORIONIC DIAMNIOTIC

This is a complication associated with monochorionic diamniotic twins. It occurs because of vascular anastomoses in the placenta.

46 A – DICHORIONIC DIAMNIOTIC

The lambda sign is chorionic tissue between the two gestation sacs. Therefore the twins will be dichorionic diamniotic.

47 C – MONOCHORIONIC MONOAMNIOTIC

The number of yolk sacs reflects the amnionicity of the pregnancy. Therefore these twins are monoamniotic.

48 C – MONOCHORIONIC MONOAMNIOTIC

Cord entanglement could only happen in a monoamniotic pregnancy.

49 A – DICHORIONIC DIAMNIOTIC

Feticide using this method can only be performed when there is no chance of vascular anastomoses between the twins, i.e. in dichorionic twins.

50 A – DICHORIONIC DIAMNIOTIC

Early splitting of one embryo results in dichorionic diamniotic twins.

51 C – MONOCHORIONIC MONOAMNIOTIC

Late splitting of one embryo results in monochorionic monoamniotic twins.

52   A – MONOCHORIONIC MONOAMNIOTIC

This is true for monochorionic monoamniotic twins.

FETAL ULTRASOUND ABNORMALITY

53   D – 47,XX+21

These are features of Down's syndrome. 1:3 fetuses with an atrioventricular septal defect will have trisomy 21.

54   D – 47,XX+21

Duodenal atresia is an abnormality associated with Down's syndrome. 1:3 fetuses with duodenal atresia will have trisomy 21. It is often seen on ultrasound in the late second or third trimester.

55   C – 47,XX+18

These are features associated with trisomy 18 (Edwards' syndrome).

56   B – 47,XX+13

Midline facial and brain abnormalities are associated with trisomy 13 (Patau's syndrome).

57   J – TRIPLOIDY

These are features of triploidy.

58   F – MECKEL–GRUBER

These are the features of Meckel–Gruber syndrome.

59   C – 47,XX+18

These features are associated with trisomy 18 (Edwards' syndrome).

DRUGS IN PREGNANCY

60   A – CLEFT PALATE

Cleft palate is associated with phenytoin treatment.

61   H – REDUCED LIQUOR VOLUME

Indometacin reduces fetal renal blood flow and this can lead to a reduction in liquor volume.

62   D – NASAL HYPOPLASIA AND CHONDRODYSPLASIA PUNCTATA

Nasal hypoplasia and chondrodysplasia punctata are features of warfarin embryopathy. Of children born to women exposed to warfarin in the first trimester, 15–25% may develop hydrocephaly, microcephaly, malformations of the vertebral bodies, intrauterine growth restriction and neurodevelopmental delay.

63   H – REDUCED LIQUOR VOLUME

ACE inhibitors affect fetal renal function causing oligohydramnios and skull defects.

64   C – ENLARGED RIGHT ATRIUM AND TRICUSPID REGURGITATION

Ebstein's anomaly is associated with lithium therapy in pregnancy, and 1–12% of offspring of mothers exposed to lithium may be affected. Exposure in late pregnancy has been associated with polyhydramnios and diabetes insipidus.

LATE TERMINATION OF PREGNANCY

65   D – POTASSIUM CHLORIDE FETICIDE PRIOR TO INDUCTION OF LABOUR WITH MIFEPRISTONE AND PROSTAGLANDINS

Termination of pregnancy is permitted at any gestation if there is a significant risk of serious handicap. After 22+0 weeks' gestation measures must be taken to ensure that the fetus is not born alive, unless the baby would die in the immediate neonatal period from its abnormality. In this case the baby would die from prematurity rather than trisomy 18, and therefore feticide is necessary.

66   C – INDUCTION OF LABOUR WITH MIFEPRISTONE AND PROSTAGLANDINS

In this case the baby would die in the immediate neonatal period from anencephaly and therefore feticide is not necessary.

67   F – SELECTIVE FETICIDE USING UMBILICAL CORD OCCLUSION

As there is the possibility of vascular anastomosis in a monochorionic twin, placenta cord occlusion is necessary. If potassium chloride is used, there is the chance that it could cross into the circulation of the unaffected twin and that twin could die. Also if one twin in a monochorionic pair demises there is the chance of death of the co-twin due to the vascular anastomosis.

68   A – CANNOT OFFER TERMINATION UNDER CLAUSE E

Absence of a hand does not fulfil the criteria of serious handicap. Serious handicap implies that individuals would need considerable support with activities of daily living (such as washing and eating) and would be unlikely to live independently. Individuals with one hand can live full and independent lives.

69   A – CANNOT OFFER TERMINATION UNDER CLAUSE E

Although the circumstances are very sad this does not fulfil the legal criteria for termination of pregnancy.

SPINAL ANATOMY

70   C – L1,L2

The spinal cord terminates at the level of the lower border of the L1 vertebra.

71   G – S2,S3

The subarachnoid space terminates at the level of the lower border of the S2 vertebra.

72   I – T10

The umbilicus represents dermatome T10.

73   K – T4

The T4 dermatome is at the level of the nipples. This ensures a peritoneal block.

74   A – C5,C6

75   F – S1

76   H – S2,S3,S4

This enables the use of the forceps and administration of an episiotomy without pain sensation for the patient.

EMERGENCY DRUG TREATMENT

77   J – EPHEDRINE 3 MG

Ephedrine is a vasoconstrictor and can be given in 3 mg boluses to restore normotension.

78   B – ADRENALINE 0.5 ML OF 1:1000

The scenario is of an anaphylactic reaction which should be treated with 500 µg of adrenaline.

79   C – ADRENALINE 1 MG

The woman has pulseless electrical activity. This is a non-shockable rhythm and adrenaline 1 mg should be the first drug to be given.

80   H – ATROPINE 0.3 MG

As a pulse is present, a 0.3 mg dose of atropine should be used.

ANTENATAL PROBLEMS

81   M – REPEAT DOPPLER AND LIQUOR IN 2 DAYS AND ADMINISTER STEROIDS

The woman has the risk factor of gestational diabetes and subsequently has developed intrauterine growth retardation (IUGR). Although delivery is not imminent, steroids and a repeat Doppler in 2 days is warranted.

82   L – REPEAT DOPPLER AND LIQUOR IN 1 WEEK

There are signs of IUGR and in addition the history of a small baby. Thus more intensive monitoring is required. As the Doppler is normal, a scan sooner is not required.

83   J – INDUCTION OF LABOUR WITHIN 24 HOURS WITH PROSTAGLANDIN

Cholestasis is managed differently by different individuals, however in view of the patient being term and the biochemical abnormalities, induction of labour is an acceptable course of action. The risk of fetal demise in cholestasis is reported to be up to 3%. Monitoring is not beneficial and does not predict intrauterine fetal death. Ursodeoxycholic acid has been shown to improve the symptoms of cholestasis, but there is no conclusive evidence that it improves fetal outcome.

84   I – INDUCTION OF LABOUR WITH SYNTOCINON

The differential diagnosis is chorioamnionitis or meconium liquor. The latter is more likely as the patient is afebrile and there is no evidence of fetal tachycardia. The safest option despite the low Bishop's score is Syntocinon rather than alprostadil (Prostin) in view of the possibility of fetal distress. Of women presenting with meconium staining of liquor, there is associated fetal distress in 33%.

85   G – DELIVER BY EMERGENCY CAESAREAN SECTION

An abnormal trace in the presence of suspected IUGR warrants caesarean section. It is unlikely that there will be time to administer two doses of steroids. The bleeding may also be indicative of the presence of an abruption. Despite the prematurity, caesarean section is the correct option.

MANAGEMENT ON THE DELIVERY SUITE

86   L – MONITOR ON DELIVERY SUITE FOR FETAL OR MATERNAL COMPROMISE

This woman has a diagnosis of an abruption or a placental edge bleed. At present there is no fetal or maternal compromise. In view of the gestation the correct management would be to administer steroids and to observe for any compromise which would indicate a caesarean section. Prolonged PV bleeding would also warrant caesarean section.

87   E – ADMIT TO ANTENATAL WARD AND REVIEW THE NEXT DAY REGARDING MODE OF DELIVERY

One has to question the reason for induction and whether it is really required at 38 weeks. However, a decision has been made to deliver the baby and although the ideal management may be option D, in this scenario

Answers: Obstetrics

the correct management would be admission to the ward followed by a decision regarding the mode of delivery. Also, in view of the irregular tightenings this patient should be admitted to the ward, in case of spontaneous rupture of membranes and cord prolapse or rupture of the uterus.

88 L – MONITOR ON DELIVERY SUITE FOR FETAL OR MATERNAL COMPROMISE

This woman has a diagnosis of bleeding with placenta praevia. There is no fetal or maternal compromise. In the absence of urgency, awaiting fetal or maternal compromise is the correct option. Also the scenario occurs at 6 am so the consultant would not be in the hospital. It is wise to have a senior obstetrician in attendance when performing the caesarean section.

BREAST CANCER IN PREGNANCY

89 E – ADVISE TO WAIT 2–3 YEARS AFTER TREATMENT OF BREAST CANCER

The current RCOG advice is to wait 2–3 years after cessation of treatment. There is no evidence of worsening of prognosis of breast cancer following pregnancy. Tamoxifen use has been associated with side effects similar to diethylstilbestrol exposure and increased intrauterine fetal death in rodents.

90 A – 1 IN 3000

The current incidence of breast cancer in pregnancy is 1 in 3000 and the incidence of cervical and ovarian cancer is 1 in 1200–10 000 and 1 in 5000–18 000, respectively.

MALPRESENTATION

91 D – EXTERNAL CEPHALIC VERSION

Evidence-based medicine would support offering external cephalic version to a woman not in labour and found to have a breech presentation at term. Approximately 50% of fetuses can be converted to a cephalic presentation with approximately 50% of those reverting back to breech.

92 E – INTERNAL PODALIC VERSION

The second twin requires urgent delivery. Internal podalic version would avoid LSCS and expedite delivery. If it was unsuccessful, LSCS could be done. In current practice this can be done in theatre, depending on the experience of the obstetrician.

93   A – DO NOTHING AND REVIEW IN ANTENATAL CLINIC

It is likely that this fetus will revert spontaneously at this gestation. Rechecking the presentation at term would be appropriate management.

94   F – VAGINAL BREECH DELIVERY

Delivery appears imminent. Rushing to perform an emergency LSCS could put the mother at risk and could result in a difficult LSCS. Good progress in labour is a favourable sign of an uncomplicated breech delivery.

95   F – VAGINAL BREECH DELIVERY

The outcome for this fetus is extremely poor irrespective of mode of delivery. LSCS would jeopardise the mother, could necessitate a classic caesarean section and is not likely to improve the outcome for the fetus. Under these circumstances, it is possible that continuous monitoring would also be inappropriate.

ANTENATAL MANAGEMENT

96   E – EXPECTANT MANAGEMENT AND INDUCE ONLY IF POST-MATURE

The current green top guideline from the RCOG suggests that patients who remain continent after a previous third or fourth degree tear should be allowed to proceed with a vaginal delivery. Therefore, option E is the correct answer. Any patient who has problems with faecal function should be offered a caesarean section at term.

97   E – EXPECTANT MANAGEMENT AND INDUCE ONLY IF POST-MATURE

Ultrasound scanning for estimated fetal weight has a 10–15% leeway. Because the head is engaged and there are no other problems this woman should have expectant management. Induction of labour for larger babies carries the risks of complications which may increase the need for surgical delivery. There is currently no conclusive evidence that induction of labour at or just before term will increase the possibility of a vaginal delivery.

98 E – EXPECTANT MANAGEMENT AND INDUCE ONLY IF POST-MATURE

As this woman's previous baby had mild shoulder dystocia that required only primary manoeuvres, expectant management and induction if post-mature is the correct option.

99 I – INDUCTION OF LABOUR AT 40 WEEKS

In view of the otherwise uncomplicated pregnancy and the relatively favourable cervix, induction of labour is the best option. The risks of problems in a macrosomic infant include shoulder dystocia. There should be close monitoring of good progress in labour and a low threshold for intervention. Approximately 50% of pregnant women with diabetes will end up with a caesarean section. Some may argue a caesarean section at term is best option, however there is no evidence that this is a better option.

100 C – ELECTIVE CAESAREAN SECTION AT TERM

Secondary manoeuvres were required to deliver this woman's last child, and therefore her present baby is at high risk of shoulder dystocia. On balance a caesarean section performed electively at term is the best option.

101 E – EXPECTANT MANAGEMENT AND INDUCE ONLY IF POST-MATURE

The management of all the scenarios in this EMQ are subject to the individual obstetrician's preference. There is no adequate evidence to support the management decision in many of these scenarios. Some doctors want to avoid the use of dinoprostone when overdue at term, but this woman is quite adamant to try for a normal delivery. After appropriate counselling with regards to uterine rupture, the use of prostaglandins to induce labour is quite acceptable.

OBSTETRIC COLLAPSE

102 G – PLACENTA PRAEVIA

The choice of option for this scenario is between G and H. The clue in the question is the high head at term in a primigravida, which is in keeping with placenta praevia rather than a diagnosis of abruption.

103 A – AMNIOTIC FLUID EMBOLISM

The absence of signs suggestive of other conditions makes amniotic fluid embolism the most likely. The risk of maternal mortality in these women is approximately 50%. Traditionally, the diagnosis has been made by the pathologist who may find fetal squames in the lungs. On average there are between 8 and 10 histologically confirmed diagnoses in deceased patients.

104 N – THROMBOEMBOLISM

The history of possible recurrent miscarriage, pain in the left loin and sudden death point to pulmonary embolism. Women with recurrent miscarriage may benefit from aspirin with or without heparin in the antenatal period.

105 H – PLACENTAL ABRUPTION

The history of possible IUGR, bleeding, irregular tightenings and CTG abnormality all point to the possibility of placental abruption. If asked, the correct management here is caesarean section.

106 J – PRIMARY POSTPARTUM HAEMORRHAGE

A gift question! The time scale makes this a primary postpartum haemorrhage.

107 P – UTERINE RUPTURE

The first sign of uterine rupture is usually CTG abnormalities. On complete rupture the engaged head may become abdominal.

ACUTE PRESENTATION IN OBSTETRICS

108 E – FIBROID UTERUS

The only answer that fits the signs and symptoms is a fibroid uterus undergoing red degeneration.

109 O – UTERINE INVERSION

Sudden unexplained collapse in the absence of excessive bleeding should alert the clinician to the possibility of uterine inversion. However, this is extremely rare and usually associated with mismanagement of the third stage of labour. Vaginal examination will confirm the diagnosis.

Answers: Obstetrics

110 C – ATONIC UTERUS

The most common cause, and hence the most likely cause here, of primary postpartum haemorrhage is an atonic uterus, whether or not the patient has had an instrumental delivery. Other causes of postpartum haemorrhage are trauma, retained tissue and thrombophilia.

111 M – TORSION OF AN OVARIAN CYST

Out of the possible options torsion is the most likely. Urinary tract infections do not usually cause rebound tenderness. Ovarian torsion presents with tachycardia, raised temperature and a raised white cell count.

112 P – VASA PRAEVIA

Vasa praevia is the most likely diagnosis in view of the recent ARM and bradycardia. Prompt delivery may save the baby, but he or she may be severely compromised and anaemic.

LABOUR WARD MANAGEMENT

113 A – ADMINISTER EPIDURAL

Despite the understandable wishes of the patient, the long latent phase is now over and rapid progression to full dilatation is expected. An epidural can bring some relief to the patient, particularly after a long induction. Considerate counselling and explanation can work wonders.

114 J – DELIVER BY NEVILLE–BARNES FORCEPS

A difficult decision to make, but the least trauma to the mother would be caused by a forceps delivery as opposed to a caesarean section. The advantage of forceps delivery over the vacuum is that there would be little or no maternal effort. A caesarean section would be relatively more difficult with the head on the perineum.

115 F – CALL FOR SENIOR HELP

Two people are better than one. This baby certainly needs to be delivered and involvement of senior support may sway the woman's decision. This of course is in an ideal situation when senior support is at hand.

116 J – DELIVER BY NEVILLE–BARNES FORCEPS

Due to the relative prematurity, the forceps is less likely to cause significant trauma than vacuum.

MANAGEMENT OF THE SECOND STAGE OF LABOUR

117 P – START SYNTOCINON

This patient is failing to progress in the second stage. There is no obvious fetal distress. For an assisted delivery it is imperative to have regular moderate/strong contractions. Therefore administration of Syntocinon to stimulate contractions prior to delivery is warranted.

118 L – INCREASE RATE OF SYNTOCINON

In a primigravida it is relatively safe to increase the rate of Syntocinon particularly if she is only contracting every 5 minutes. Repeat assessment in approximately 2 hours would demonstrate whether suitable progress has occurred.

119 K – EXTERNAL CEPHALIC VERSION

In the absence of fetal distress, external cephalic version may allow delivery of the second twin by changing the presentation to cephalic. Rupture of membranes at this stage could lead to a cord prolapse and necessitate an emergency caesarean section.

POSTPARTUM HAEMORRHAGE

120 I – CROSS-MATCH 4–6 UNITS OF BLOOD

The initial management is to cross-match blood as this is likely to take longer than a senior arriving (presuming that they live at a distance of within 30 minutes of the hospital).

121 J – EXAMINE UNDER GENERAL ANAESTHESIA

Examination under anaesthesia is the next step in order to stem the bleeding. While in theatre Hemabate can be administered. Removal of placental tissue will hopefully stem the blood loss, but if it does not have the desired effect an intrauterine balloon may be of benefit.

122 B – ADMINISTER ERGOMETRINE WITH OXYTOCIN (SYNTOMETRINE)

Repeating the dose of Syntometrine is simple and easily administered as long as the woman is not hypertensive. Syntocinon infusion may also be started and intrauterine clots evacuated.

PROBLEMS IN THE PUERPERIUM

123 E – ENDOMETRITIS

The history and examination all point to endometritis. Retained products of conception comes a close second. Prolonged labour and instrumental delivery both increase the incidence of endometritis.

124 N – THROMBOEMBOLISM

The most likely cause is pulmonary embolus. Emergency caesarean section after a prolonged labour and the symptoms appearing at day 4 suggest embolisation of a deep vein thrombus.

125 A – ATONIC UTERUS

The most likely cause of postpartum haemorrhage is atony of the uterus. Retained products of conception following a caesarean section are highly unlikely.

126 H – MASTITIS

Absence of fluctuation makes a breast abscess unlikely. Postpartum pyrexia of unknown origin should always involve examination of the breasts.

GYNAECOLOGY

AMBIGUOUS GENITALIA AND PRIMARY AMENORRHOEA

127   J – MEYER–ROKITANSKY–KÖSTER–HAUSER SYNDROME

Forty per cent of girls with Meyer–Rokitansky–Köster–Hauser syndrome have renal abnormalities with 15% having major abnormalities. It is the second most common cause of primary amenorrhoea after Turner's syndrome (XO).

128   E – GONADAL DYSGENESIS

The presence of a uterus in a 46,XY karyotype is particular to gonadal dysgenesis. Möllerian-inhibiting factor (MIF) is not produced and therefore the uterus may develop.

129   A – ANDROGEN INSENSITIVITY

In androgen insensitivity (testicular feminisation) MIF is produced, but testosterone cannot exert its influence on hair growth. Breast development is usually normal.

130   O – TURNER'S SYNDROME

Girls with Turner's syndrome often present to the general practitioner because of their short stature, but it is not until failure of menstruation that investigations lead to the diagnosis.

131   I – KALLMANN'S SYNDROME

Anosmia is the clue here. These girls usually have normal stature.

SEXUAL HEALTH

132   B – *CALYMMATOBACTERIUM GRANULOMATIS*

Calymmatobacterium granulomatis is endemic in Africa, and also among the aboriginal population of Australia. The condition is known as donovanosis. Treatment with antibiotics often leads to resolution of the ulcer, which helps to discriminate from vulval cancer.

133 G – HERPES SIMPLEX

Patients with primary genital herpes often present with urinary retention and pain in the perineum. Aciclovir may be useful in reducing the length and alleviating the pain of primary genital herpes.

134 L – *TRICHOMONAS VAGINALIS*

The most likely culprit is *Trichomonas vaginalis*.

135 D – *CHLAMYDIA TRACHOMATIS*

Both gonococcus and *Chlamydia* can cause Fitz–Hugh–Curtis peri-hepatic adhesions. *Chlamydia* is more common so this is the correct answer as the question asked for the most likely cause.

136 F – GROUP B HAEMOLYTIC STREPTOCOCCUS

A relatively straightforward question owing to the previous history of Group B haemolytic streptococcus septicaemia. Antibiotic prophylaxis in labour is essential with a history of previous neonatal septicaemia.

137 L – *TRICHOMONAS VAGINALIS*

Florid *Trichomonas* infections are often associated with red lesions on the cervix and vagina.

CONTRACEPTION

138 E – IMPLANON IMPLANT

Many of the options listed may be appropriate in such a scenario; however, one must balance the risks with the failure rate. High-dose progesterone and oestrogens are absolute contraindications, but adequate contraception is essential as pregnancy has a high risk of maternal mortality. In a 16-year-old Implanon is more desirable than a levonorgestrel intrauterine system as the uterus may not have fully developed. The patient must be counselled with regard to abnormal vaginal bleeding that occurs with the use of Implanon.

139 B – COPPER IUCD

A previous failure, consideration of her age and marital status and in the absence of menorrhagia, the IUCD is the best choice.

140   I – MALE CONTRACEPTION

On balance, in patient with so many risks and in a relationship where future fertility is not likely to be an issue, vasectomy is the wisest option. Of course, people do not always choose the most appropriate option.

141   D – GYNEFIX IUCD

The GyneFix IUCD is designed for the nulliparous patient. The use of condoms should also be advised to avoid sexually transmitted infection.

EMERGENCY GYNAECOLOGY (1)

142   N – RETROVERTED UTERUS

In the absence of genital and urinary infection, retroversion of the uterus is the most likely answer. This most commonly presents at 14 weeks' gestation and catheterisation and conservative management are usually sufficient.

143   A – APPENDICITIS

The most likely diagnoses here are appendicitis and PID. PID is usually bilateral thus leaving appendicitis. In addition, diarrhoea may indicate appendicitis.

144   E – ECTOPIC PREGNANCY

This most likely represents an ectopic pregnancy with formation of a pseudosac.

145   K – OVARIAN TORSION

The grid-iron scar is that of an appendicectomy. Therefore, ovarian torsion is the most likely diagnosis.

EMERGENCY GYNAECOLOGY (2)

146   K – REFER TO REGIONAL CENTRE FOR FURTHER TREATMENT

Routine repeat evacuation is not warranted in gestational trophoblastic disease unless either requested by a regional centre or if haemorrhaging. Any problems in the management of gestational trophoblastic disease should be discussed with the regional centre.

147 C – CHECK β-HCG IN 48 HOURS

The correct management would be to repeat the hCG in 48 hours as long as the patient is stable. Ultrasound should be able to identify an intrauterine pregnancy when the hCG level is between 1000 IU and 1500 IU.

148 H – LAPAROTOMY AND SALPINGECTOMY

Some would question the use of laparoscopic surgery here. However, on balance, for the majority laparotomy is the mainstay for a ruptured ectopic pregnancy in a haemodynamically unstable patient.

149 K – REFER TO REGIONAL CENTRE FOR FURTHER TREATMENT

This is most probably persistent gestational trophoblastic disease so referral to the regional centre is advised. Persistent gestational trophoblastic disease can occur after any pregnancy. After miscarriage, normal pregnancy or ectopic pregnancy the prognosis is worse mainly due to a delay in diagnosis.

150 M – REPEAT ULTRASOUND SCAN IN 7–10 DAYS

In a stable patient in early pregnancy a repeat ultrasound scan is better than repeating an hCG level in 48 hours as this is more likely to give a diagnosis.

151 A – ADMINISTER SYNTOMETRINE INTRAMUSCULARLY

The initial management would be to stem the bleeding. Intramuscular Syntometrine is quick and easy to administer.

CLINICAL GYNAECOLOGICAL PROBLEMS

152 L – GONOCOCCAL INFECTION

Infections of the peri-urethral glands of Skene lead to a pungent discharge, which is usually green. This discharge may become more apparent on vaginal examination.

153 A – ADENOMYOSIS

Adenomyosis can be exquisitely tender on bimanual examination. This condition affects approximately 1% of women. The normal pelvis suggests there is no endometriosis.

154 C – *CANDIDA* INFECTION

A simple swab can lead to the diagnosis of *Candida* infection. Steroids may make the condition worse. Misdiagnosis of vulval problems is relatively common.

155 B – BACTERIAL VAGINOSIS

Bacterial vaginosis is the most likely problem. The discharge may occasionally improve and then worsen. Treatment with metronidazole may improve the symptoms temporarily, but in the long term this treatement can be unrewarding.

ABNORMAL BLEEDING IN GYNAECOLOGY

156 F – *CHLAMYDIA* INFECTION

Initially the use of depot injections may lead to abnormal bleeding, but in an established user it is most probably because of *Chlamydia* infection. Abnormal bleeding only due to the depot injection is more commonly found in women with a raised BMI. Any woman using depot injections who presents with abnormal bleeding should have triple swabs taken.

157 K – ENDOMETRIOSIS

These are cardinal symptoms of endometriosis. Dyspareunia, dysmenorrhoea, dyschezia (pain on opening bowels) and dysuria may all be associated with endometriosis.

158 K – ENDOMETRIOSIS

The differential diagnosis is between ovarian cancer and endometriosis. In this woman's age group endometriosis is more likely. PID is also a possibility, but is not there in the list of options. However, investigation by laparoscopy would provide the diagnosis.

159 G – DYSFUNCTIONAL UTERINE BLEEDING

Dysfunctional uterine bleeding is a diagnosis of exclusion. Endometrial malignancy is rare in this age group especially without risk factors.

GYNAECOLOGICAL INVESTIGATION

160 E – ENDOMETRIAL PIPELLE
Endometrial Pipelle is the most useful investigation as this is likely to give a histological diagnosis. Hysteroscopy may also be useful but will not give a histological diagnosis.

161 F – FSH, LH AND OESTRADIOL
The only part missing in the history is 'hot flushes'. The single most useful diagnosis would be a hormonal profile. A hysteroscopy may be a useful investigation, but alone may not give a diagnosis.

162 C – CT SCAN
A CT scan is useful not only to discriminate the nature of the cyst, but also to alert the clinician to the possibility of lymph nodes. It also aids in staging.

163 B – CERVICAL SMEAR
Women with HIV infection are more likely to develop cervical cancer, as the history suggests here. A cervical smear should give a diagnosis. Any immunocompromised woman should have annual smears.

164 I – MRI
MRI is the most useful investigation for staging purposes. This will give the depth of invasion and also indicate the presence of abnormal lymph nodes.

UROGYNAECOLOGY

165 H – URETHRAL DIVERTICULUM
Urethral diverticula are becoming more common and affect 3% of the female population. The increase in incidence is thought to be due to the increasing incidence of sexually transmitted diseases. The clue in the history is the post-micturition dribble.

166 K – VESICO-VAGINAL FISTULA
Trauma from the cone biopsy may lead to the development of a vesico-vaginal fistula. Incontinence is unlikely to leave a person constantly damp, especially at this woman's age.

167 G – OVERFLOW INCONTINENCE

Overflow incontinence after epidural anaesthesia is potentially preventable by inserting an indwelling catheter until normal bladder sensation returns. Mismanagement of the bladder can lead to problems that are difficult to rectify.

168 B – DETRUSOR OVERACTIVITY

Detrusor instability may lead to the symptoms of urge incontinence and nocturia.

169 E – MIXED STRESS INCONTINENCE AND DETRUSOR INSTABILITY

The most likely answer here is a urinary tract infection. Exclusion of urinary tract infection is an essential first-line step in any patient who complains of urinary symptoms.

ENDOCRINOLOGY

170 F – PITUITARY ADENOMA

The raised prolactin makes the diagnosis of a pituitary microadenoma obvious.

171 E – MENOPAUSE

Menopause is the most likely diagnosis. Of course if the patient was below 40 years of age then it may represent premature ovarian failure.

172 C – HYPOGONADOTROPHIC HYPOGONADISM

Hypogonadotrophic hypogonadism due to either a low BMI or excessive exercise is the most likely diagnosis from the list of options.

173 G – POLYCYSTIC OVARIAN DISEASE

The inverse ratio of LH and FSH and the slightly elevated testosterone point to PCOS. The testosterone level is also marginally elevated.

INFERTILITY

174 E – ENDOMETRIOSIS
The history is suggestive of endometriosis. Male factor infertility is unlikely as her partner has one child from a previous marriage (presuming the child is his).

175 H – HYPOGONADOTROPHIC HYPOGONADISM
The low BMI suggests the diagnosis. Hypogonadotrophic hypogonadism may occur in anorexia and also in athletes.

176 K – PCOS
The irregularity of the cycle and the high incidence of PCOS of about 20% help to make the diagnosis. Her BMI is also raised.

177 L – PREMATURE OVARIAN FAILURE
This unfortunate woman has premature ovarian failure. Such women should be counselled about the use of hormone replacement therapy, sometimes best given in the form of the oral contraceptive pill. In addition, there is a rare possibility of ovulation and therefore barrier methods of contraception should be advised if the oral contraceptive pill has not been prescribed.

INFERTILITY INVESTIGATION

178 I – SEMEN ANALYSIS
Smoking or working in a smoky environment may lead to a reduction in sperm count. In the absence of any female infertility, male factor infertility should point the couple in the right direction.

179 H – RUBELLA ANTIBODY TITRE
Strictly, this patient does not as yet have a diagnosis of infertility as she has not been trying to conceive for 1 year. A rubella antibody test, however, would be useful.

180 E – HYSTEROSCOPY
A hysteroscopy to rule out Asherman's syndrome after the evacuation would probably be the single most useful test. Vigorous curettage in the

puerperium may lead to the production of intrauterine synechiae or scar tissue.

181 F – LAPAROSCOPY AND DYE PERTURBATION

This history suggests tubal damage. The normal menstrual cycle suggests ovulation and the previous pregnancy suggests that her partner has a normal semen analysis.

CONSENT GUIDELINES

182 D – 1 IN 4000

All these can be found on the RCOG consent guidelines produced by the professional standards committee.

183 K – 5%

184 K –5%

CONSENT GUIDELINES FOR DIAGNOSTIC LAPAROSCOPY AND VAGINAL HYSTERECTOMY

185 H – 5 IN 100 000

186 F – 2 IN 1000

187 E – 2 IN 100

SURGICAL COMPLICATIONS

188 K – SMALL-BOWEL OBSTRUCTION

This is a classic history of symptoms that occur 11–14 days after the original laparotomy. Paralytic ileus is unlikely at this stage. If symptoms do not settle with conservative management a repeat laparotomy is necessary.

189 F – MYOCARDIAL INFARCTION

Acute LBBB, unlike RBBB, is a sign of myocardial infarction and is nearly always due to a pathological cause.

190 A – BLEEDING REQUIRING RESUTURING

Bleeding requiring resuturing usually occurs in the hours immediately following surgery. Bleeding after 24 hours usually results in a self-limiting haematoma that can be managed conservatively.

191 B – BOWEL PERFORATION

Pain requiring readmission to hospital following a laparoscopy should always alert the clinician of possible bowel perforation and should not be ignored. Thorough investigation and involvement of other disciplines are warranted.

LAPAROSCOPIC ENTRY TECHNIQUES

192 B – 0.5%

Bowel adhesions to the anterior abdominal wall are found in 0.5% of patients without prior surgery, 20% with a previous Pfannenstiel incision and 50% with a previous midline incision.

193 J – REDUCES INCIDENCE OF VASCULAR TRAUMA ONLY

Open laparoscopy will reduce the incidence of vascular trauma and is advocated in patients with an anticipated complicated entry due to previous surgery. Current evidence suggests that bowel injury is not reduced, but is more readily identified.

DRUG THERAPY IN GYNAECOLOGY

194 P – TRANEXAMIC ACID

Tranexamic acid should not be prescribed to patients who have had previous thromboembolic disease as it may increase the risk of deep vein thrombosis.

195 N – METRONIDAZOLE

Routine treatment for *Trichomonas vaginalis.*

196 J – DULOXETINE

Duloxetine is a selective serotonin and noradrenaline reuptake inhibitor, and increases the tone of the rhabdosphincter.

197 B – AZITHROMYCIN

Failure of treatment of *Chlamydia* may indicate poor compliance. Therefore a single dose of azithromycin may be more suitable. However, re-infection is a possibility.

198 F – CLINDAMYCIN

Clindamycin is an adequate replacement for patients allergic to penicillin.

GYNAECOLOGICAL ONCOLOGY – CERVIX

199 G – CYTOLOGY

Borderline cervical smears account for 7% of all cervical smear results. They are therefore very common. Around 10% of women with borderline smear results will actually have histologically proved high-grade pre-cancer. The UK guidance is that women with persistent borderline smears should be referred for colposcopy. Therefore this woman should have a repeat smear after 6 months.

200 I – LOOP EXCISION OF THE TRANSFORMATION ZONE

Young women who have incomplete excision of CIN3 are generally conservatively managed. However, retrospective studies have demonstrated that women over 45 years of age are at increase risk of cervical cancer, and UK policy is to repeat the loop excision in such a scenario.

201 J – MRI

MRI is the optimal imaging technique to stage cervical disease. It is excellent at determining size and local invasion of disease, and is also good at determining lymph node size.

202 B – CHEMO-RADIATION

The UK recommendations are that women with bulky stage 1b disease should be treated with primary chemo-radiation. There is a high risk of metastatic lymph node involvement and incomplete excision of the primary tumour if surgery is performed.

203 O – TRACHELECTOMY

In young women with early (1b) disease who wish to preserve their fertility radical trachelectomy preserves uterine function.

Answers: Gynaecology

ENDOMETRIAL CANCER

204 M – TAMOXIFEN

Tamoxifen usage is associated with a 2–7-fold increase in incidence of endometrioid adenocarcinoma, papillary serous carcinoma and carcinosarcomas of the uterus. This risk may continue for up to 10 years following cessation of treatment.

205 I – MRI

MRI has the advantage over CT scan as it can determine the extent of disease in the myometrium. Both CT and MRI are good at determining lymph node enlargement.

206 D – COMBINED CONTRACEPTIVE PILL

Women with polycystic ovaries and oligomenorrhoea are at increased risk of developing endometrial cancer. If they do not want to conceive, the combined contraceptive pill will give them a regular withdrawal bleed and protect the endometrium.

VULVAL NEOPLASIA

207 O – VULVAL BIOPSY

All women with persistent vulval symptoms, particularly ulceration, should have a vulval biopsy to exclude invasive disease.

208 L – SUPERFICIAL AND DEEP ILIO-FEMORAL NODE DISSECTION

Staging lymph node dissection should include the superficial and deep iliofemoral nodes.

209 J – SENTINEL LYMPH NODE BIOPSY

Sentinel lymph node biopsy aims to identify the first node a tumour drains to. If this can be identified, and it is histologically normal, formal iliofemoral dissection is not performed. This is because there is a high chance that further nodes will be normal, and thus sparing the patient of surgery with high morbidity.

VULVAL DISEASE

210 H – PSORIASIS

Generalised psoriasis can affect the vulva. Women with a previous history of psoriasis with a vulval lesion might have psoriasis. It is therefore imperative to examine the skin in other areas to establish a clinical diagnosis.

211 E – HIDRADENITIS SUPPURATIVA

Hidradenitis suppurativa is more common in Afro-Caribbean women. It is associated with thickening of the labia majora and indurated nodules.

212 A – CANDIDAL VULVOVAGINOSIS

Vulval and vaginal candidiasis is more common in women with diabetes. In women with a history of recurrent thrush this disease should be excluded.

OVARIAN NEOPLASIA

213 I – OVULATION INDUCTION

Ovulation induction leads to an increase in epithelial damage in the ovary. Women who have had Clomid therapy or *in-vitro* fertilisation (IVF) cycles are more at risk of developing epithelial tumours of the ovary.

214 B – CEA

Krukenberg's tumours are often associated with metastatic bowel or stomach tumours. Therefore CEA might be elevated.

215 O – SPECIFICITY

Specificity is a measure of a test's ability to predict normality. If a test has a poor specificity, then the false-positive rate might be high.

CERVICAL CANCER AND DYSKARYOSIS

216 D – 95%

The prognosis for early cervical cancer is extremely good and in the order of 95%.

217 I – HPV TYPES 6 AND 11
HPV types 6 and 11 are associated with genital warts.

218 C – 70%
The sensitivity of screening cytology is around 70%.

219 M – PRE-TERM LABOUR
Retrospective controlled studies have clearly demonstrated a higher incidence of pre-term labour, and cervical incompetence after knife cone biopsy.

GESTATIONAL TROPHOBLASTIC DISEASE

220 J – HONG KONG
Molar pregnancy and associated choriocarcinoma is commoner in the Far East.

221 I – HCG
Persistent molar pregnancy or choriocarcinoma is associated with elevated levels of hCG.

FAMILIAL AND DRUG-RELATED RISK OF CANCER

222 D – ENDOMETRIAL CANCER
Women with this autosomal dominant condition have a 20% risk of developing endometrial cancer.

223 F – OVARIAN CANCER
Women with the *BRCA1* gene are at risk of both ovarian and breast cancer. Breast cancer is not strictly classed as a gynaecological cancer in the UK.

224 H – VULVAL CANCER
Women with vulval dystrophy have a higher risk of developing vulval cancer.

GYNAECOLOGICAL ONCOLOGY SURGERY

225 K – VAGINAL HYSTERECTOMY

Women with cervical glandular intraepithelial neoplasia are at risk of developing invasive adenocarcinoma. If an excisional biopsy demonstrates pre-invasive disease only, and excision is incomplete then it is safe to perform a vaginal hysterectomy.

226 G – OBTURATOR NODES

Pelvic lymphadenectomy should include obturator, external and internal pelvic lymph node chains.

227 D – INFRA-COLIC OMENTECTOMY

A staging laparotomy for ovarian cancer should include infra-colic omentectomy.

CERVICAL SCREENING AND HPV

228 H – LOOP EXCISION

A type 3 transformation zone suggests that the upper limit of the transformation zone is deep in the cervical canal. Therefore this disease should not be treated by ablative treatment – it should be treated only by excision.

229 G – LIQUID-BASED CYTOLOGY

Liquid-based cytology has reduced the inadequate smear rate from 12% to less than 1%.

230 E – IMIQUIMOD

Imiquimod is a potent immune response modifier and stimulates the immune system against HPV infections.

STATISTICS (1)

231 A – HIGH SENSITIVITY

A test that has a very low false-negative rate has high sensitivity.

232 E – LOW THRESHOLD

A low threshold for a test reduces its false-negative rate; conversely a high threshold leads to high false negatives and therefore low sensitivity.

233 H – RECEIVER OPERATOR CHARACTERISTIC CURVE

A receiver operator characteristic curve (ROC) demonstrates test performance at different thresholds.

STATISTICS (2)

234 I – SECONDARY ANALYSIS

A study that only analyses the outcomes of patients who complete treatment is described as a secondary analysis.

235 F – POWER CALCULATION

The power of a study is determined by the sample size and the difference between the magnitudes of difference between the outcomes. This needs to be determined so that sample size can be estimated.

236 J – SYSTEMATIC REVIEW

A comprehensive review of all the evidence, conducted with scientific methods, is likely to give the most reliable evidence.

237 C – INTENTION TO TREAT ANALYSIS

A study that includes all the patients initially recruited in the final analysis is called an intention to treat analysis.

STATISTICS (3)

238 B – 8%

$32/400 = 0.08$ or 8%.

239 F – 75%

Sensitivity is the probability that the test (abdominal palpation) will correctly diagnose a true case (breech presentation on scan) – $24/32=0.75$ or 75%.

240 G – 87%

Specificity is the probability of correctly classifying a non-case – 320/368=0.87 or 87%.

241 D – 33%

The positive predictive value is the probability that a case with a positive result (palpates breech) really does have a positive result (is breech on scan) – 24/72=0.33 or 33%.

ETHICAL AND MEDICO-LEGAL PRINCIPLES

242 B – BATTERY

Performing a procedure without consent on a patient who is deemed competent despite being stressed and in pain leaves the doctor who has performed the procedure vulnerable to a charge of battery.

243 H – NEGLIGENCE

Failure of the doctor to respond to a midwife's call when there is possible fetal distress amounts to negligence.

244 G – FRASER (GILLICK) COMPETENCE

When offering termination of pregnancy or giving contraceptive advice it is important to establish whether the girl is competent under the Fraser guidelines (also known as Gillick competence). It is important to clarify that she understands the advice; she cannot be persuaded to inform her parents; her best interest requires the practitioner to perform the procedure.

245 E – CONFIDENTIALITY

Permission of the patient must be sought prior to disclosing any information to a third party.

246 K – VERACITY

Being truthful to the patient, veracity, is the principle being disregarded here. Confidentiality is not in question as you have not disclosed the information to the family.

247 J – PATERNALISM

When making a decision for the patient without giving any options or involving the patient in the decision is a paternalistic approach.

248 A – AUTONOMY

When a patient is deemed competent, it is her right to refuse treatment despite the consequences. This is the principle of autonomy. The doctor must then try to offer an acceptable alternative.

249 C – BENEFICENCE

Doctors may make decisions and act in the patient's best interest when informed consent is not available in situations where there is a risk of serious harm or death. The patient must not have made a previous directive regarding refusal of treatments.

250 E – CONFIDENTIALITY

Disclosing results to a third party without the permission of the patient is breaching patient confidentiality.

INDEX

abdominal pain 86, 108, 123, 143
ACE inhibitors 63
aciclovir 19, 23, 133
adenomyosis 153
adnexal masses, bilateral 158
adrenaline 78, 79
advance directive 249
amenorrhoea 130–131, 175, 177
amniocentesis 33, 35
amniotic fluid embolism 103
anaphylactic reaction 78
androgen insensitivity 129
anencephaly 32, 65
anosmia 131
antenatal management 96–101
antenatal problems 81–85
antenatal screening 30–36
anti-D prophylaxis 42, 43
anti-hypertensives in pregnancy 12–15
antibiotics, adverse reaction 78
appendicitis 143
ascites 158, 162
Asherman's syndrome 180
aspirin, antenatal 104
atenolol, during pregnancy 15
atrioventricular septal defect 53
atropine 80
autonomy 248
azithromycin 197

battery 242
beneficence 249
beta-blockers, risk of IUGR 15
betamethasone 154
biceps tendon reflex 74
bile acids 83
biophysical profile 2
bipolar disorder 64
bleeding
    requiring resuturing 190
    see also vaginal bleeding

blood, cross-matching 120
blood pressure, checking 9
blood transfusion 184, 187, 248
bowel
    adhesions 192
    perforation 191
bradycardia 112, 114
BRCA1 gene, mutations 223
breast cancer 89–90, 204, 223
breast development 129, 130
breasts, tender/erythematous 126
breech presentation 91, 93, 94, 95

CA125 162
caesarean section
    complications 120
    elective 100, 248
    emergency 85, 113, 114, 123, 124
calcium gluconate 17, 18
Calymmatobacterium granulomatis 132
cancer, familial and drug-related
    risk 222–224
Candida infection 154, 212
captopril 63
carcinoembryonic antigen (CEA) 214
cardiac arrest 80
cataracts, congenital 24
cerebral palsy 243
cervical cancer 163, 164, 199–203, 216–219
cervical intraepithelial neoplasia (CIN)
    219, 220, 225
cervical screening/smear
    163, 199, 218, 228–229
cervix
    barrel-shaped 164
    incompetence after conisation 219
    long and closed 85, 86, 97
chemo-radiation 202
chest pain, sudden-onset 189
child, termination of pregnancy 244
child abuse, resulting in pregnancy 69

Index

Chlamydia infection   135, 156, 197
cholestasis   83
chondrodysplasia punctata   62
choriocarcinoma   220
chorion villus biopsy   30, 36
choroid plexus cysts   34, 60
chromosomal analysis *see* karyotype
cleft palate   60
clindamycin   198
clinical gynaecological problems   152–155
clinical practice, reliable evidence   236
Clomid therapy   213
colposcopy, referral   199
condoms   141
cone biopsy   166, 219
confidentiality   245, 246, 250
congenital heart disease   34, 60, 63, 64
congenital varicella syndrome   24
consent guidelines   182–184, 185–187
contraception   138–141
contraceptive pill   10, 139, 206
convulsions   11
CT scan, for ovarian cysts   162
cystic fibrosis   25, 26
cytology   199
cytomegalovirus   20, 22

danazol   196
deep vein thrombosis   140, 194
delivery mode, decision   88
delivery suite, management   86–88
Depo-Provera   156
depression   14
dermatomes   72, 73
detrusor overactivity   168, 169
diabetes
    and chronic vulval irritation   212
    in pregnancy   5–8, 81
    type 1   99
diabetes insipidus   64
diarrhoea   143
diazepam   17
dichorionic pregnancy   44, 46, 49, 50, 119
dietary modification   7
dinoprostone   101
diuretics   12
donovanosis   132
Doppler investigations   2, 37, 81, 82

double bubble, on ultrasound scan   54
Down's syndrome   30, 33, 53, 54
drugs
    for emergency treatment   77–80
    in gynaecology   194–198
    in pregnancy   60–64
ductus venosus, Doppler   2
Duloxetine   196
duodenal atresia   54
dyschezia   157, 174
dysmenorrhoea   157
dyspareunia   153, 157, 165, 174
dysuria   157

Ebstein's anomaly   64
ectopic pregnancy   144, 148, 149, 181, 245
Eisenmenger's complex   138
embryo, cleavage   50, 51
enalapril, contraindicated in pregnancy   10
encephalocele   58
endocrinology   170–173
endometrial cancer   204–206, 222
endometrial cavity, sac   144
endometrial Pipelle   160
endometriosis   157, 158, 174
endometritis   123
ephedrine   77
epidural anaesthesia   77, 113
epilepsy, drugs in pregnancy   60
ethical and medico-legal principles   242–250
examination under anaesthesia   121
exomphalos   34
expectant management   86, 87, 96
external cephalic version   90, 119

false negatives   232
family, disclosing information to   250
fertility, conserving   203
fetal anaemia   1, 37
fetal bradycardia   77
fetal head
    direct occiput anterior (DOA)   115, 116
    left occiput transverse (LOT)   117
    right occiput transverse (ROT)   118
    strawberry-shaped, on ultrasound
      scan   55

Index

fetal imperfections, not justifying termination 68
fetal movements, absent 16
fetal renal function 63
fetal size 2, 57
fetal tachycardia 107, 243
fetal ultrasound abnormality 53–59
fetal wellbeing 1–4
feticide 49, 65, 67
fever 19, 95
fibroids 108, 247
fingers, overlapping, on ultrasound scan 60
fists, clenched, on ultrasound scan 60
Fitz–Hugh–Curtis peri-hepatic adhesions 135
flexion contractures 24
follicular phase endocrine profile results 170–173
forceps delivery 114, 116, 167, 242
Fraser (Gillick) competence 244

gastroschisis 4
genetics 25–29
genital warts, prophylactic vaccine 217
genitalia, ambiguous 128
gestational trophoblastic disease 146, 149, 220–221
glucagon 8
glucose tolerance test 6, 7
gonadal dysgenesis 128
gonococcal infection 152
grid iron scar 145
groin node dissection 209
growth scans 3, 4
gynaecological emergencies 142–145
gynaecological investigation 160–164
gynaecological oncology
    cervix 199–203
    surgery 225–227

haematuria 157
haemorrhage, postpartum 106, 120–122, 180, 184
Hartmann's solution, intravenous 18
hemabate 121
hepatosplenomegaly 22
hereditary non-polyposis colon cancer 222
herpes simplex 23, 133

hidradenitis suppurativa 211
holoprosencephaly 56
homocystinuria 27, 28, 29
hormonal profile 161, 170–173
human chorionic gonadotrophin (hCG) 144, 147, 221
human immunodeficiency virus (HIV) infection 163
human papillomavirus (HPV) 217, 230
hydrocephaly 62
hydropic fetus 21
hypertension in pregnancy 9–11
hypoglycaemia 8
hypogonadotrophic hypogonadism 172, 174
hypotension 77, 148
hysterectomy
    total abdominal 182, 183, 188
    vaginal 187, 225
hysteroscopy 180

imaging techniques 201
    see also CT, MRI
imiquimod 230
Implanon implant 138
in-vitro fertilisation (IVF), risk of ovarian tumours 213
indometacin 61
induction of labour
    in late termination 65, 66
    for macrosomia 99
    with oxytocin 84, 113
    for post-maturity 96, 97, 98, 101, 112
    with prostaglandins 83, 101
infections in pregnancy 19–24
infertility 174–177
    investigations 178–181
infra-colic omentectomy 227
instrumental delivery, refusal 115
insulin 5, 7
insurance company report 245
intention to treat analysis 237
internal podalic version 91
intrauterine contraceptive devices (IUCDs) 139, 141
intrauterine growth retardation (IUGR) 4, 15, 62, 81, 82, 85
intravenous access 16
itching of palms and soles 83

Index

Jarisch–Herxheimer reaction 21
Jehovah's witnesses 248

Kallmann's syndrome 131
karyotypes
    46XX 127
    46XY 128, 129
    47XX+13 56
    47XX+18 55, 59
    47XX+21 53, 54
Kell positive 37
kidneys
    absent 127
    multicystic 59
Kleihauer's test 38–41
knife conisation 166, 219
Krukenberg's tumour 214

labetalol 13
labia majora, chronic painful nodules 211
labour ward management 113–116
lambda sign 46
laparoscopy 181, 185–186, 191–193
laparotomy 148, 245, 246
left bundle branch block (LBBB) 189
left iliac fossa pain 111
liquid-based cytology 229
liquor, abnormalities 3, 4, 62, 63, 84, 95, 112
lithium 64
lochia, offensive and heavy 123
loin tenderness, bilateral 142
loop excision 200, 228
lymph nodes 208, 226

McRoberts' position 98
macrosomia 7, 87
magnesium 11, 16, 17, 18, 74
malaise 19
male contraception 140, 141
male factor infertility 178
malpresentation 91–95
mastitis 126
Meckel–Gruber syndrome 58
membranes, rupture 84, 95, 112
menopause 171
menorrhagia 153, 157, 194

menstruation, irregular 161
methyldopa 13, 14
metronidazole 155, 195
Meyer–Rokitansky–Köster–Hauser
    syndrome 127
microcephaly 21, 22, 62
middle cerebral artery, peak systolic velocity
    measurement 1
midline abnormalities 56
mifepristone 65, 66
Möllerian-inhibiting factor (MIF) 128, 129
molar pregnancy 146, 220
MRI, for staging 164, 201, 205
myalgia 19
myocardial infarction 189

nasal hypoplasia 62
negligence 243
neural tube defect 66
neurodevelopmental delay 62
Neville–Barnes forceps delivery 114, 116
nifedipine 10
nocturia 168
normotension, restoring 77

obstetric collapse 102–107
obstetrics, acute presentation 108–112
obturator lymph nodes 226
oligohydramnios 59, 63
oligomenorrhoea 206
oliguria, following delivery 18
oophorectomy, complications 190
ovarian cancer 213–215, 223, 227
ovarian cysts 111, 145, 147, 162
ovarian failure, premature 171, 177
ovulation induction 213
oxytocin 113, 117, 118, 121, 122, 151

paternalism 247
patient
    best interest 249
    non-disclosure of diagnosis 246, 250
pelvic inflammatory disease (PID) 143
pelvic lymphadenectomy 226
pelvic pain 104, 135, 158, 165, 191
penicillin allergy 198

peri-urethral glands of Skene 152
perinatal mortality, risk 52
petechial rash 22
pethidine 113
phenytoin 17, 60
pituitary adenoma 170
placenta
    abruption 85, 86, 105
    large 21, 57
    vascular anastomoses 45, 67
placenta praevia 87, 88, 102
polycystic ovary disease 173, 176, 206
polyhydramnios 7, 54, 64
polymerase chain reaction (PCR) 20, 31
positive predictive value 241
post-micturition dribbling 165
power of a study, calculation 235
pre-eclampsia 11, 16–18
pre-term labour, increased incidence 219
prevalence, calculating 238
prostaglandins 65, 66, 83
prosthetic heart valve 62
proteinuria, monitoring 9
proteinuric hypertension 16, 17, 18
pruritus vulvae 154, 210
pseudosac 144
psoriasis 210
pubic hair, absence 130
pudendal nerve 76
puerperal problems 123–126
pulmonary embolism 104, 124
pulmonary oedema 248
pulseless electrical activity 79

rash 19, 210
receiver operator characteristic (ROC) curve 233
referral to regional centre 146, 149
renal abnormalities 127
retained products of conception 146, 180
rhesus disease 1, 31, 38–42
right atrium, enlarged 64
right fornix, tenderness 143
right iliac fossa pain 145
ring pessary 169
rocker bottom feet 55
rubella antibody titre 179

salpingectomy, laparoscopic 149
sample size, assessing 235
sandal gap 53
sciatica, in pregnancy 61, 75
screening tests 231, 233
second stage of labour, management 117–119
secondary analysis 234
semen analysis 178
senior support, calling for 115
sensitivity of a test 231, 232, 239
sentinel lymph node biopsy 209
septicaemia 136
serious handicap, defining 68
sexual health 132–137, 165
short stature 130
shoulder dystocia 98, 100
skull defects 63
small-bowel obstruction 188
specificity of a test 215, 240
spinal anaesthetic 72, 73
spinal anatomy 70–76
statistics 231–233, 234–237, 238–241
strawberry spots, cervix and vagina 137
streptococcus, group B haemolytic 136, 198
subarachnoid space 71
suprapubic tenderness 169
surgical complications 188–191
symphysis–fundal height 96, 105
Syntocinon/Syntometrine *see* oxytocin
syphilis, congenital 21
systematic review 236

talipes, bilateral 34, 55
tamoxifen 89, 204
tear, fourth degree 96
termination of pregnancy
    in a child 244
    late 65–69
testicular feminisation 129
beta-thalassaemia 36
thiazide diuretics 12
threshold, low 232
thromboembolism 104, 124
thrush 212
trachelectomy 203
tranexamic acid 194
translocations 35
transverse presentation 92, 119

Index

treatment, refusal 248, 249
Treponema pallidum 21
trials, design 234, 237
Trichomonas vaginalis 134, 137, 195
tricuspid regurgitation 64
triploidy 57
trisomy 13 (Patau's syndrome) 56
trisomy 18 (Edwards' syndrome)
34, 55, 59, 65
trisomy 21 53, 54
tubal damage 181
tumour markers 214, 221
Turner's syndrome 130
twin delivery 92
twin pregnancy 44–52, 67, 119
twin to twin transfusion syndrome 3, 45

ultrasound scan, repeat 150
umbilical cord 48, 67
ureteric injury, risk 182, 183
urethral diverticulum 165
urinary incontinence 166–169
urinary retention 23, 133, 142
urinary tract infections 165, 169
urodynamics assessment 196
urogynaecology 165–169
ursodeoxycholic acid 83
uterovaginal prolapse 169
uterus
    absent 127, 129
    at level of umbilicus 121, 125
    atonic 110, 125
    bleeding, dysfunctional 159
    cancer risk 204
    evacuation 146
    fibroid 108
    inversion 109
    large for dates 108
    retroversion 142
    rupture 101, 107, 109

vacuum extraction 110
vaginal bleeding
    abnormal 156–159
    abruption 105
    after evacuation of uterus 146
    inter-menstrual 163

management 85, 86, 88, 102, 151
    painless 147, 150
    persistent 221
    post-coital 163
    postmenopausal 160, 232
    postpartum 106, 110
vaginal delivery, preference for 101
vaginal discharge
84, 134, 136, 143, 152, 155
vaginosis, bacterial 155
varicella zoster (chickenpox) 19, 24
vasa praevia 112
vasectomy 140
ventriculomegaly 20
veracity 246
vertebral body malformations 62
vesico-vaginal fistula 166
viral infections 20
vulva
    biopsy 207
    bleeding 132
    cancer 207–209, 224
    disease 210–212
    dystrophy, and cancer risk 224
    pain/irritation 133, 154, 207, 210, 212
    ulceration 23, 132, 133, 207
    warts 230
vulvovaginosis 212

warfarin 62

yolk sacs 47